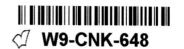
Post-Traumatic Stress Disorder

Jerry Cott '86

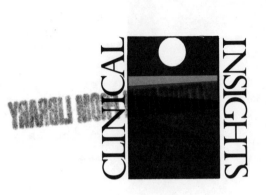

Post-Traumatic Stress Disorder: Psychological and Biological Sequelae

Edited by
BESSEL A. VAN DER KOLK, MD

Lecturer in Psychiatry, Harvard Medical School
at Massachusetts Mental Health Center
and Cambridge Hospital

AMERICAN PSYCHIATRIC PRESS, INC.
Washington, D.C.

ABF 8471

Note: The authors have worked to ensure that all information in this book concerning drug dosages, schedules, and routes of administration is accurate at the time of publication and consistent with standards set by the U.S. Food and Drug Administration and the general medical community. As medical research and practice advance, however, therapeutic standards may change. For this reason and because human and mechanical errors sometimes occur, we recommend that readers follow the advice of a physician directly involved in their care or the care of a member of their family.

This monograph is based on material presented at the 136th Annual Meeting of the American Psychiatric Association. That meeting and this monograph are endeavors to share scientific findings and new ideas. The opinions expressed in this monograph are those of the individual authors and not necessarily those of the American Psychiatric Association.

© 1984 American Psychiatric Association

Library of Congress Cataloging in Publication Data

Main entry under title:

Post-traumatic stress disorder.

(Clinical insights)
Includes bibliographies.
1. Post-traumatic stress disorder—Complications and sequelae. 2. Post-traumatic stress disorder—Physiological aspects. 3. War neuroses—Complications and sequelae 4. Veterans—United States—Psychology. 5. Vietnamese Conflict, 1961-1975—Psychological aspects. I. van der Kolk, Bessel A. II. Series. [DNLM: 1. Stress disorders, Post-Traumatic. WM 184 P8565] RC552.P67P67 1984 616.85'21 84-6375
ISBN 0-88048-053-X (pbk.)

Printed in the U.S.A.

Contents

Contributors

HELENE BOYD, PhD

Research Fellow in Psychiatry, Veterans Administration Outpatient Clinic, Boston; and Instructor of Psychology in Psychiatry, Harvard Medical School

ELIZABETH BRETT, PhD

West Haven Veterans Administration Medical Center and Department of Psychiatry, Yale University

B. CULLEN BURRIS, MD

Albany Medical College and U.S. Veterans Administration

AUGUSTIN DE LA PENA, PhD

Chief, Clinical Psychophysiology Laboratory, Audie L. Murphy Memorial Veterans' Hospital, San Antonio

CHARLES DUCEY, PhD

Director of Training in Clinical Psychology, Cambridge Hospital; and Instructor of Psychology in Psychiatry, Harvard Medical School

M. S. GALLOPS, MPhil

Department of Sociology, Columbia University; and The Center for Policy Research, New York

MARY C. GRACE, MEd, MS

Research Associate, Department of Psychiatry, University of Cincinnati Medical School

BONNIE L. GREEN, PhD

Assistant Professor, Central Psychiatric Clinic, Department of Psychiatry, University of Cincinnati Medical School

MARK GREENBERG, PhD

Section of Neurology, New England Deaconess Hospital, Boston; and Instructor of Psychology in Psychiatry, Harvard Medical School

SUSAN GRIFFITHS, RN
U.S. Veterans Administration, Albany

LOIS KINNEY, PhD
Department of Psychology, University of Cincinnati

LAWRENCE C. KOLB, MD
Distinguished Physician, U.S. Veterans Administration, Albany

MILTON KRAMER, MD
Professor of Psychiatry and Human Behavior; and Director, Dream/Sleep Laboratory, Veterans Administration Medical Center, Jackson, Mississippi

HENRY KRYSTAL, MD
Professor of Psychiatry, Michigan State University; and Lecturer, Michigan Psychoanalytic Institute

JOHN KRYSTAL
Medical Student, Yale University School of Medicine

ROBERT S. LAUFER, PhD
Department of Sociology, Brooklyn College/Graduate Center, City University of New York; and The Center for Policy Research, New York

JACOB D. LINDY, MD
Associate Clinical Professor, Department of Psychiatry, University of Cincinnati Medical School

LAWRENCE S. SCHOEN, PhD
Assistant Director, Dream/Sleep Laboratory, Veterans Administration Medical Center, Jackson, Mississippi; and Assistant Professor of Psychology in Psychiatry, University of Mississippi Medical Center

BESSEL A. VAN DER KOLK, MD
Lecturer in Psychiatry, Harvard Medical School at Massachusetts Mental Health Center and Cambridge Hospital

Introduction

The role of psychological trauma as a precursor of mental disorders has, until recently, been a much neglected area of research in psychiatry. Since Freud abandoned his theory of actual seduction as the cause of hysteria, psychoanalysis has tended to down play the role of catastrophic psychological events on further personality development. Wars, concentration camps, and civilian disasters from time to time have inspired profound psychological works about the impact of traumatic stress (e.g., Grinker and Spiegel 1945; Lifton 1968; Krystal 1968; Erikson 1976). Only in the past decade, however, has the ubiquity and pervasiveness of post-traumatic states in psychiatry become recognized.

Two lengthy studies on the effects of civilian trauma have been particularly seminal: the work of Mardi Horowitz (1976) on the interaction between trauma and preexisting personality and on the phases of post-traumatic stress, and the studies on the disaster at Buffalo Creek (Erikson 1976). In addition, the war in Vietnam, which originally had claimed the lowest rate of psychological casualties of any American-fought war, produced a staggering number of men with post-traumatic stress disorder (PTSD). The lack of recognition of this syndrome as being on a continuum with previously described post-traumatic states initially led to the coining of a separate term: Post Vietnam Syndrome. Among the many outstanding contributors to the understanding of PTSD in Vietnam veterans are Figley (1978), Hendin (1981), Shatan (1977), Fox (1974), Williams (1980), Wilson (1979), and Haley (1974), several of whom were Vietnam veterans themselves.

When the syndrome of post-traumatic stress disorder was incorporated into the third edition of the *Diagnostic and Statistical Manual of Mental Disorders* (DSM-III) (American Psychiatric Association 1980), particularly because of the efforts of clinicians working with Vietnam veterans, the criteria for the syndrome were essentially the same as those described by Abraham Kardiner (1941) on the basis of his observations of World War I (WWI) veterans. Studies on children and adults in both war and peace have confirmed the accuracy of Kardiner's observations, namely that the psychological effects of trauma consist of an alternation between hyperreactivity (startle reactions, explosive outbursts of anger) and recurrent intrusive recollections of the trauma (flashbacks, nightmares, hypermnesia) on the one hand, and on the other hand, a warding off of these phenomena, with psychic numbing, constriction of affect and social functioning, as well as a profound loss of a sense of control over one's destiny.

The existence of cultural and temporal modifiers in the expression of PTSD is exemplified by the fact that although conversion reactions are omnipresent in descriptions of "shell shocked" WWI soldiers and psychosomatic sequelae are frequently mentioned in WWII veterans, neither of these appears to be common in Vietnam veterans, where behavior disorders are described more frequently. It is likely that catastrophic psychic trauma, particularly in childhood, may contribute to such diverse psychiatric disturbances as psychosomatic conditions, chronic pain syndromes, and certain character disorders, including borderline conditions, in addition to the core symptomatology of adult PTSD. The precise interaction between trauma, constitutional factors, level of personality development, cultural factors, and the ultimate expression in the form of altered affect, behavior, pain perception, and somatic functioning remains an unexplored territory.

Since the first descriptions of psychological trauma, observers have recognized that post-traumatic states have both a pronounced psychological and a physiological expression. Freud (1920) suggested that traumatic neurosis entails a "physical fixation" to psychic trauma. Kardiner and Spiegel (1947) asserted that traumatic neurosis is a "physioneurosis" with "a lasting perceptual heightening of stimuli signaling threat." Under the partial influence of Lawrence Kolb (Chapter 6) and various sleep researchers (Chapters 5 and 7) both here and abroad, a renewed interest in the physiological aspects of PTSD has surfaced recently. The laboratory model of inescapable shock (Chapter 8) is unique in providing an animal model of a human psychiatric syndrome, allowing for controlled measurements of behavioral, physiological, and biochemical alterations subsequent to overwhelming stress.

The question of who develops post-traumatic sequelae in response to stress remains partially unanswered. Victims of Nazi concentration camps have probably been studied with more care over a longer period of time than any other traumatized population (Krystal, Chapter 1), and it is striking to what degree many sequelae of the concentration camp experience appear to parallel those of Vietnam veterans (Chapters 1 and 2) and victims of civilian disaster (Chapters 1 and 3). Epidemiological studies of Vietnam veterans (Chapter 4) seem to confirm many earlier clinical observations, but also have come up with surprising new findings about vulnerability.

In recent years Leonore Terr's (1983) study of the Chowchilla schoolbus kidnapping has provided fascinating new data about the development and course of PTSD in children. While she found that the severity of post-traumatic symptoms was correlated with preexisting family pathology, lack of community bonding, and individual vulnerabilities, every one of the 25 kidnapped children continued to have manifestations of PTSD four years after the schoolbus kidnapping. Moreover, the post-traumatic symptoms were strikingly similar despite the fact that the group included children of oedipal, latency, and adolescent phases of development. She came to the conclusion that none of the children was "toughened" by the experience, that they "simply had narrowed their spheres of concern to their own rooms at night," and had lost hope to be able to affect their own future. The traumatic etiology of affective and behavioral disturbances in patients is easily overlooked—during the hyperreactive phase, the management of these patients may prove to be so challenging that they may receive a psychiatric label that denotes more the frustrations of their management team than an accurate diagnosis. During the phase of psychic numbing these patients interact little with the outside world, they tend not to ask for psychiatric help, and are more likely to be found in compensation offices and in medical consultation rooms. Outsiders who probe into the trauma are often soon identified as aggressors and victimizers. As in most aspects of PTSD, controlled treatment studies are lacking, but clinical indications are that those who find others who share their traumatic past are best able to make an affective involvement in the present. By clarifying some of the psychological and physiological issues underlying post-traumatic stress disorder we hope to contribute to a better treatment of people who suffer from its sequelae.

Bessel A. van der Kolk, M.D.

References

Erikson K: Everything in Its Path—Destruction of Community in the Buffalo Creek Flood. New York, Simon and Shuster, 1976

Figley CR: Stress Disorders Among Vietnam Veterans. New York, Brunner-Mazel, 1978

Fox RP: Narcissistic rage and the problem of combat aggression. Arch Gen Psychiatry 31:807–811, 1974

Freud S: Beyond the Pleasure Principle (1920), in Complete Psychological Works, standard ed, vol 18. Translated and edited by Strachey J. London, Hogarth Press, 1959

Grinker RR, Spiegel JP: Men Under Stress. Philadelphia, Blakiston, 1945

Haley SA: When the patient reports atrocities. Arch Gen Psychiatry 30:191–196, 1974

Hendin H, Haas AP, Singer P, et al: Meanings of combat and the development of posttraumatic stress disorder. Am J Psychiatry 138:1490–1493, 1981

Horowitz MJ: Stress Response Syndromes. New York, Jason Aronson, 1976

Kardiner A: The Traumatic Neuroses of War, in American Handbook of Psychiatry, Vol I. Edited by Arieti S. New York, Basic Books, 1941

Kardiner A, Spiegel H: War Stress and Neurotic Illness. New York, Hoeber, 1947

Krystal H: Massive Psychic Trauma. New York, International Universities Press, 1968

Lifton RJ: Death in Life: Survivors of Hiroshima. New York, Random House, 1968

Shatan CF: Bogus manhood, bogus honor: surrender and transfiguration in the US Marine Corps. Psychoanal Rev 25:335–349, 1977

Terr L: Chowchilla revisited: the effects of psychic trauma four years after a schoolbus kidnapping. Am J Psychiatry 140:1543–1550, 1983

Williams T: Psychological Adjustment of Vietnam Veterans. Disabled American Veterans Outreach Program, Washington, DC, 1980

Wilson JP: The Forgotten Warrior Project. Disabled American Veterans Association, Washington, DC, 1979

1

Psychoanalytic Views on Human Emotional Damages

Henry Krystal, M.D.

1

Psychoanalytic Views on Human Emotional Damages

. . . so low for long, they never right themselves;
You may see their trunks arching in the woods
Years afterwards, trailing their leaves on the ground . . .
——Robert Frost, Birches (1916)

The origins of psychoanalysis and modern psychiatry are intimately involved with approaches to the challenge of psychic trauma. For instance, Freud stressed the traumatic origin of hysteria in opposition to the then predominant theory of degeneracy causing neuroses. He held two different theories of trauma: the "unbearable affect" theory and the "unacceptable impulse" theory. Characteristically, he could contain diverse views and labor for years to reconcile them. He stated both of these views quite early and simultaneously (Freud 1893a, 1893b). In the unbearable experience view the *emotions* evoked by the traumatic situation were responsible for the aftereffects. The implication was that they threatened to overwhelm the psyche and in the process of trauma become strangulated. Freud (1893b, p 38) proposed that "hysterical patients suffer from incompletely abreacted psychical traumas." The unacceptable impulse theory was stated as follows:

It turns out to be a *sine qua non* for the acquisition of hysteria that an incompatability should develop between the ego and some idea presented to it (p 122); and the actual traumatic moment, then, is the one at which the incompatibility forces itself upon the ego and at which the latter decides on the repudiation of the incompatible idea. That idea is not annihilated by a repudiation of this kind, but merely repressed into the unconscious. (p 123)

Freud was able to reconcile these two conceptions of trauma only after clarifying the role of anxiety as the signal of (internal) danger. He explained that if the defensive actions—notably repression—failed, there was a mounting of the anxiety and a progression to "automatic anxiety."

The two views did have something in common from the beginning, namely their attempt to explain the circumstances under which *repression* became necessary. Thus, Freud's approaches to psychic trauma mapped out a limited territory for exploration: the kind of traumatic experiences which lead to the development of neuroses—those related to the conflicts on the phallic level of psychosexual development.

During World War I (WWI), a number of Freud's students and fellow analysts were in the ranks of physicians to the armed forces of the Central Powers. There they encountered a syndrome of acute panic that allowed for a generalization of the views of psychic trauma which were originally so narrowly defined. In 1919 Freud stated:

Some of the factors which psychoanalysis had recognized and described long before as being at work in peace time neuroses—the psychogenic origin of symptoms, the importance of *unconscious* instinctual impulses, the part played in dealing with mental conflict by the primary gain of being ill (flight into illness)—were observed to be present equally in the war neuroses and were accepted almost universally. Simmel's studies show also what successes could be achieved by treating war neurotics by the method of catharsis which, as we know, was the first step toward the psychoanalytic technique. (p 207)

The effectiveness of the "cathartic method" resulted in a reactivation of Freud's early ideas about the strangulated affects, and the need to drain them. Other methods of therapy—such as local electric shock—were also used with some success in the Vienna University Psychiatric Clinic, but the postwar suit brought by veterans accusing Wagner-Jauregg of cruelty gave Freud another chance to demonstrate the superiority of psychological treatment as contrasted to the use of "strong electric current" (Freud 1919, p 214).

The experience of World War II (WWII) did not favor the resumption of the "traumatic neurosis" model. Even when only the "war neuroses" were considered, leaving out the psychotic, characterological, psychosomatic, and addictive problems, a variety of syndromes of anxiety and operational fatigue were found, and the last word of Grinker and Spiegel (1945, p 348) was: "*Neuroses of wars* are psychoneuroses." The point being that "*after the initial blow, the pattern is internalized and repetitive according to the previous patterns of the personality.*"

Moreover, the acute, self-limited picture of traumatic neurosis as redefined by Kardiner (1941) tended to persist, and new cases were found as many as 15 years after the end of World War II, with many acute conditions becoming chronic (Archibald et al. 1962). Studies of the degree of continuing disability, sponsored by the U.S. Veterans Administration, showed that of the veterans who were judged ill at discharge (23 percent of the sample), "the overwhelming majority . . . remained unchanged 10 years later." In fact, "about 10 percent grew worse after discharge. Most of the men who were *severely* disabled were in the main men who improved after leaving service" (Brill and Beebe 1955, p 144). Moreover, the follow-up ten years later showed essentially no difference in the status of the veterans based on the mode of treatment of the original episode; that is, whether they received "A—no more than rest and sedation; B—individual therapy; or C—hospital routine. The degree of maladjustment and disturbance and follow-up correlated best with the degree of success or failure in adjustment *prior* to service." Still, "groups devoid of significant psychiatric defects at entry contributed about 35 percent of all among World War II admissions for all psychiatric diagnoses except psychosis or mental deficiency. . . . In 1944 they constituted half the admissions for psychoneurosis" (Brill and Beebe 1955, p 333).

Statistical studies reviewing the experience of WWII went beyond the simplistic impressions of the handful of analytic observers of WWI. Thus, it was shown that psychological tolerance was subject to much variation. For instance, soldiers with psychiatric admissions prior to combat broke down more rapidly than those without such prior admissions. Furthermore, "men with courts-martial for AWOL prior to entering combat broke down more rapidly than the other men" (Beebe and Appel 1958, p 147).

Special problems were observed in the postwar era in follow-ups of ex-prisoners of war. The mortality and morbidity of ex-prisoners of war, particularly of Japanese camps, was found to be significantly elevated during the first five years after liberation. This included all causes of death—even accidents (Cohen and Cooper 1954). "The exceedingly high death rate during imprisonment seemed to persist at and shortly after liberation, then diminished rapidly within the first period of observation leaving an apparently persistent residual mortality excess . . . " (p 19). As for the persisting disabilities, "they were also ten times higher in the ex-prisoners of the Japanese camps compared to those of the European detention, and fifty times higher than in the veterans who were not imprisoned. The same group had twice the rate of psychoneuroses . . . and other neuropsychiatric conditions" (p 39). However, the rate of somatic conditions—such as gastritis, enteritis, and functional intestinal disorders—was equal among both groups of ex-prisoners and four to five times higher than in the rest of the veterans.

In my follow-up observations I have struggled in vain to fit the survivors of the Nazi Holocaust into the "classical" psychoanalytic concepts of psychic trauma. I concluded that our observations simply could not be understood in terms of the economic view of traumatization, nor in terms of Freud's other definition of trauma, namely repression (Krystal 1968c). The symptoms which I listed at that time were problems of persisting unmanageable aggression, "affect lameness," and certain characterological observations:

"many of the male survivors tend to be permanently inhibited in their ability for sexual initiative and potency in a manner reminding us of the ethological concept of the 'defeated' male" (p 3). I further observed that there were "severe inhibitions of intellectual function, memory, and interest . . . " (p 3), which I thought represented, in part, overcompliance with the Nazi attempt to reduce the Jews to a dumb slave role. I wondered about symptom pictures which were called "break in the life-line" and "collapse of the personality," and how we could account for such states as "the individual who has lost his ability to enjoy life, to trust others or to display any initiative" (p 5). I wrestled with observations of survivors whose problems included a disturbance in affect expression and communication, and in whom the degree of anxiety and tenseness experienced prevented them from communicating anything except demands or anger (p 7).

I found that not the intensity, but the *meaning* of an experience posed the challenge and generated the affective response (Krystal 1970). Accordingly, I proposed a revision of the concept of the "stimulus barrier" from a passive barrier against impinging excitation to the totality of the apparatus involved in perception, registration, evaluation, and other components of information processing. As I stated at the time, " . . . the stimulus barrier is conceptualized actively as the total of the ego's protection against traumatization. Indeed, the effectiveness of the stimulus barrier is also influenced by intrasystemic tensions; problems of guilt and instinctual impulses may be considered predispositions to traumatization" (pp 1–2).

The "economic" conceptions of psychic trauma proved to be untenable in the light of my further observations such as postliberation psychosis, and the exceedingly high rate of psychosomatic diseases and characterological blocking of assertive and sexual functions (Krystal 1970, p 25). In some people this appeared to be a continuation of submission and aftereffects of confrontation with death which led to a destruction of basic trust, of a feeling of security, and of loss of belief in the general benevolence and causality of the world (p 24).

It became clear to me that psychic trauma could not be

understood in terms of the intensity of stimuli, but rather that we had to account for the psychic reality of the individual, and how that person interpreted and reacted to the experience (Krystal 1970). Thus, all the memories and the nature of self, object, and world representations would be involved in the shaping of the impact of a potentially traumatic experience. Further, I returned to the role of affects in traumas and came to see *affect tolerance* as being a major factor in what Freud tried to account for abstractly in terms of the conception of the stimulus barrier.

In a significant book on psychic trauma edited by Furst in 1967, Anna Freud, Solnit, Kris, and Furst repeatedly made the point that the term "psychic trauma" was used so carelessly in psychoanalytic writing that it was in danger of becoming useless. Furst (1967) felt that the outcome of trauma could be judged by the relative degree of success in mastering the traumatic stimulus, but that the "relationship of trauma to psychopathology is obligatory; it is implicit in the traumatic event itself. Whether or not the pathology *persists* will depend on post-traumatic developments. . . . The traumatic neuroses appear to substantiate Freud's view that while individuals differ in their degree of susceptibility to trauma, a limit exists in every case beyond which even the most efficacious stimulus barrier will fail" (p 20). The contributions of these researchers provided a setting for the reconsideration of the traumatic process. However, two elements still had to be provided: (1) a genetic study of affects and (2) a more thorough exploration of affect tolerance.

AFFECT AND TRAUMA

The Genetic View of Affects

Infantile affective responses can be best understood as affect precursors. They represent general and unmodulated reactions on a physiological level. The most conspicuous patterns are the state of quiescence or well-being and the distress pattern. A third pattern, the cataleptic response, disappears in the human after two months (Papousek and Papousek 1975), but it is important to keep this response in mind in reference to the "freezing" response patterns which we will encounter in the adult catastrophic patterns. The developmental lines of emotions to be taken into consideration are differentiation, verbalization, and desomatization.

In the process of maturation, emotions become more specific, and by verbalization we can pinpoint their nature more precisely. We can, for instance, identify different shades and nuances of shame such as embarrassment, chagrin, humiliation, mortification and so on. In this way, affects become useful as a source of information to us. Conversely, when there is regression, i.e., a loss of differentiation and desomatization, affects manifest themselves in a physical and nonspecific way. One may say that these infantile responses are totally psychosomatic in that, like a psychosomatic disease, they consist of physiological responses; the infant's response to distress takes a global form, characterized by total body involvement and by automatic responses. The painful affects still remain undifferentiated. In addition, the child's autonomic nervous system is so labile that affect can be transformed into pain instantaneously, e.g., anxiety into colic. Under regressive circumstances in adulthood, pain may once again become part of affective responses. This phenomenon is quite common in post-traumatic states, and a history of trauma should be suspected in pain-prone personalities.

Physiological (prepsychological) distress states mobilize so much pain and painful affect that they can be considered the forerunners of mortal dread, not fear of dying but an enormous, overwhelming, deadly anxiety. Perhaps this dread is what Klein (1946) called "psychotic anxiety," linking it with the ideation of "falling to bits." This feeling is unbearable and is the thing that causes—or, more properly, is the first part of—the traumatic process. It initiates a series of unconscious pathogenic reactions that represent the trauma syndrome. Extraordinary traumatization morbidly reinforces the commonly occurring biotraumata resulting from the normally occurring frustrations and separations. When this occurs, the reaction to danger becomes permanently excessive (Stern 1968a, 1968b).

The Ability to Utilize Affects as Signals

While signal anxiety is the alerting affect par excellence, all affects function as signals. Schur (1955) has pointed out that desomatization and verbalization are involved in affect maturation, and verbalization becomes a means of controlling and avoiding intense somatic, stressful responses. In contrast, undifferentiated affect precursors are not utilizable as signals. These are mostly somatic, vague, uncontrollable ("all or nothing") responses; their cognitive aspects are primary process and pregenitally dominated drive derivatives. The development of affect differentiation and desomatization take place in the context of the mother–child relationship. The good mothering parent takes pride in discerning the early differentiation in the vocalizing of the infant, and, being able to recognize a need, to fulfill it instantly. In this fashion he or she promotes or rewards the process of differentiation.

Individuals who have regressed in regard to affects, and those whose affect and development have been arrested are in danger of becoming overwhelmed with their responses and may have to block them completely (Krystal 1970). Traumatization in infancy and early childhood interferes with the separation of painful affects into largely verbalized and desomatized feelings of anxiety, depression, sadness, grief, shame, and so on.

Affect Tolerance

Working with certain personality disturbances convinced me that traumatization in childhood resulted in a lifelong dread of affects, and a warding off of affectivity. I became convinced that helping these patients improve their affect tolerance was a necessary preliminary phase of the treatment (Krystal 1970).

Zetzel's (1949, 1955) classical papers have established the necessity to tolerate anxiety and depression for emotional growth. The capability to handle emotions adaptively depends on the intensity and duration of the affects, and on the external and internal resources available to modulate affective experience. Like the affects themselves, patterns of affect tolerance are derived from identification with the parental love-objects. The identification is mainly with the benign mother who allows the child to experience the feeling to the intensity which the child can handle, but who interferes before it becomes overwhelming. Zetzel (1949) has pointed out that in persons whose previous self-esteem has not been contingent on absence of subjective anxiety, depressive responses are, as a rule, temporary and reversible.

The manner in which an individual experiences, evaluates, and responds to affects becomes the key to the understanding of many clinical phenomena. Fear of one's emotions and post-traumatic residuals of significant intensity tend to make one experience affects as the return of the infantile trauma state, or as the herald of the dreaded "doomsday reaction." Extreme fears of one's own affects make one vulnerable to experiencing a situation as catastrophic (Krystal 1974).

ADULT CATASTROPHIC TRAUMA

Two different kinds of psychiatric emergencies relate to emotions. One consists of a panic resulting from the fear of the magical powers of one's wishes. This fear is most commonly related to the dread of one's aggression. The other kind of emergency is related to affect tolerance. This, too, involves a panic, but the danger here is to become overwhelmed with one's emotions. Instead of being able to use them as information, one becomes terrified of the physiological (expressive) element of the emotion. This frequently results in the establishment of a vicious cycle, which magnifies and perpetuates the problem (Krystal 1982b).

When one comes to the conclusion that one is facing inescapable, unmodifiable peril, the affective pattern changes from an activating signal of preventable danger, i.e., "anxiety," to the "catatonoid reaction" (Krystal 1978a). This emotional shift may be considered the initiation of the traumatic state. It actually involves a surrender pattern that is universal throughout the animal kingdom (Richter 1957; Seligman 1975). Briefly, it consists of a paralysis of initiative, followed by varying degrees of immobilization leading to automatic obedience. At the same time there is a numbing process by which all affective and pain responses are blocked, leading to what Minkowski (1946) called "affective anesthesia."

Lifton has extended this idea to "psychic closing off" (1968). The broader conception is useful because the next aspect of the traumatic process is one in which there is progressive constriction of the cognitive processes of perception and conscious registration, including memory formation, recall, and problem solving (Krystal 1978a). Finally, just a mere vestige of self-observing functions is preserved (Petty TA: Personal Communication, 1975). This process may culminate in psychogenic death (Krystal 1978a, 1982b). It has been demonstrated (Richter 1957; Seligman 1975; Krystal 1978a) that this surrender pattern is universal in the animal kingdom and that it is a potential self-destruct mechanism. Animals of all degrees of complexity have been shown to die when merely restrained (Krystal 1982b). Psychogenic death in humans may be more common than currently suspected. On the other hand, it is possible for this process to stay at the point where a degree of psychic closing off has been accomplished that permits a certain automatonlike behavior which is necessary for survival in situations of subjugation such as prison and concentration camps (Krystal 1968a; Krystal and Niederland 1971).

Our follow-up studies (Krystal and Niederland 1968) show a continuation of depressive affect as well as depressive lifestyles in the majority of survivors. Seligman's (1975) review of animal studies also shows a continuation of patterns of submission, helplessness, and what one may call the equivalent of depressive and masochistic patterns in animals who have been subjected to severe abuse in situations of total helplessness, and even in their offspring.

Caplan (1981) has pointed out that the harmful effects of stress are modified by the cognitive guidance and emotional support that a particular setting and peer group provides. I found that in the catastrophic trauma state the speed and extent of the deterioration of ego functions will be determined by a number of factors such as the availability of group support (Krystall 1978a). When this group support fails and the individual concludes that the situation is both unbearable and unmodifiable, the deterioration becomes rapid. The ability to tolerate affects has special application under stress. The "emergency affects" are characterized by their dysphoric nature and a high degree of arousal. Hyperstimulation at first improves performance, but after a point, there is a deterioration. The point at which performance falls, however, is an individual variable. Individuals who have not been overwhelmed before have a lower physiological arousal and a better tolerance of states of high activiation (Krystal 1982–1983). Individuals with a history of psychic trauma show a physiological hyperreactivity which is part of their hypervigilance and tendency to startle, and they are prone to an early deterioration of performance. Because they are liable to expect the return of the traumatic state, they also have a tendency to panic. Conversely, familiarity and comfort with a situation ensure longer effective performance.

Horowitz (1976) has provided a model for dealing with the aftereffects of the untoward event, and/or with those situations that leave a person and his environment substantially changed. After the initial affective response, conscious registration of knowledge is handled by a partial denial of the implication of the situation. A numbing state afforded by denial is disturbed by the recurrent intrusive reappearance of the new perception in the conscious sphere. This keeps disrupting the denial and results in a renewal of affective activation. The cognitive and affective response persists as briefly as possible and is terminated by denial. There is a period of rest. Soon, the ideas intrude themselves again upon consciousness, repeating the whole cycle, which may be considered the working through process, which goes on to the completion of the work of mastery (p 56).

The process of mourning is, in fact, the process of mastering the loss, even if it is only the (temporary) loss of the illusion of invulnerability. One of the challenges in understanding catastrophic responses is to study them while simultaneously maintaining a psychologic and a biologic view of the processes. The report by Bartmeier and others (1946) reviewed the process of becoming a war casualty. The manifestations of incipient failure to maintain mastery and keep the stress within tolerable limits were first registered by irritability, hypersensitiveness, disturbances in sleep, startle reactions, and hyperreactivity to minor stimuli with increasing involuntary self-protective motor responses. Next there was a tendency to withdraw into a brooding attempt to flatten one's emotions by whatever means available including drugs, isolation, and a general loss of interest in comrades, food, letters from home, and even one's welfare. There was increasing confusion, impaired judgment, and increasing indecision. About the same time, observable problems related to the physiological components of emotion such as tremors, vomiting, and diarrhea may appear. If no help was given at this time, the confusion, irritability, and physical instability would grow to the point of reckless, incoherent, and wild behavior. Some soldiers showed catatonoid withdrawal or excitement that could lead to psychogenic death. However, at this point an outburst of rage or at least some motor activity usually occurred.

The importance of the shift to cataleptic responses as a challenge to the management of mass disasters is becoming increasingly clear (Dill 1954; Allerton 1964). Tyhurst (1951) found that 10 to 25 percent of the people involved in a disaster became stunned and immobile (indicating to me the onset of a catatonoid reaction). Studies to assess the impact of airline disasters showed that as many as half of the victims would go into a state of "panic inaction" (Johnson 1970). This is part of the rationale for the management of large groups in emergencies in a manner which is designed to prevent helpless surrender. (For a review see Krystal 1978a.) Although the passengers on a vehicle may realize that something is wrong, the crew will do its best through information to keep the general mood from becoming overwhelming. Similarly, the question of morale management in an army or in an entire population pertains to keeping the affective responses within a tolerable range.

THE AFTEREFFECTS OF CATASTROPHIC TRAUMA

At the point that a person feels that catastrophe is inevitable and uncontrollable, the affective state changes from anxiety (the affect signal of preventable danger) to the catatonoid reaction and the progression of various blocking responses. These responses are basically a continuation of the direct aftereffects beyond the period of the actual emergency.

The Recognition and Submission to Unavoidable Danger

An assumption of safety is the basis of all of our behavior patterns, including some of the most important personality traits. This (illusory) sense of security permits normal functioning. In the wake of the breakdown of the feeling of security, some individuals cannot return to the previous personality type, but assume submissive "slavelike" personalities and become incapable of assertive behavior (Krystal 1968a, 1978a) or display chronic anxiety, including paranoid states.

Studies of disasters, such as the Buffalo Creek flood, showed that the destruction of the community resulted in serious and long-lasting handicaps to its members (Erikson 1976), who were unable to function without the usual supports. The apathetic, stuporous state of people in acute emergency situations, sometimes referred to as the "disaster syndrome" (Wolfenstein 1957), may be the common sign of the loss of normal orienting responses and the onset of surrender patterns that accompanies it. The continuation of the breakdown of either the feeling of security or of the ability to utilize community supports for one's function seriously interferes with the resumption of normal life patterns.

The Surrender Pattern

When actual surrender to an external enemy or intolerable situation has taken place, shame about this surrender may either be experienced consciously or defended against in one of a number of ways. At the same time, there may be an inability to assert oneself, which actually represents a continuation of the surrender behavior.

Catatonoid Reaction as a Primal Depression

Niederland (1961, 1968, 1981) has stressed that chronic, recurrent depression was part of the symptom picture. These reactions cover "the whole spectrum from masochistic character changes to psychotic depression" (1968, p 313). Most of these depressions are not diagnosed as such, but manifest themselves as a life style of despair and commonly in physical symptoms such as chronic tiredness, weakness, and lack of resistance to illnesses. In our work with the survivors of the Holocaust, we tended to emphasize the link between these depressive reactions and the problems of guilt, particularly relevant to issues of survivorship. However, problems of depression are part of the post-traumatic picture and not limited to the survivors of genocide (Krystal 1978b).

In the surrender, in a state of total helplessness, pain stops (both physical and emotional) and a feeling of tragic sadness is experienced. In my paper on the hedonic aspect of emotions (Krystal 1981), I pointed out that there was clinical evidence of unconscious diminution of the quality of pleasure as well as of gratification. In post-traumatic states, there is a very high incidence of anhedonia, as well as attachment to painful feelings as a source of unconscious gratification (Krystal 1978a, 1981). This change in the hedonic self-regulatory system is made up of both anatomical and physiological components, involving inter alia polypeptide neurotransmitters (Snyder 1980). Animal studies on "learned helplessness," i.e., exposure to unavoidable suffering, has produced the same results, which last for a lifetime and sometimes are even transmitted to their offspring (Seligman 1975).

Affective Blocking

Affective blocking was the earliest aftereffect of traumatization reported by Minkowski (1946). In his early observations of survivors of concentration camps, he related an affective anesthesia. The same observation was made by many other investigators, including Lifton (1968) and Niederland (1961). Related to this blocking of the conscious registration of painful affects is the concurrent alexithymia, the inability to discriminate between specific feeling states, or to describe the cognitive or localizing aspects of emotions.

Alexithymia

Observations about the high frequency of psychosomatic diseases in survivors of Nazi persecution have been very consistent (Bastiaans 1957; Niederland 1961; Krystal and Niederland 1968). Similarly, there are many well-documented studies of the exceedingly high incidence of psychosomatic diseases in veterans, particularly after WWII.

It appears that the high incidence of psychosomatic diseases in posttraumatic states is related to the nature of the trauma. My colleague and I found that while the overall incidence of psychosomatic disease was 30 percent in survivors in general, in those who were under 20 years of age during the persecutions, the rate went up to 70 percent (Krystal and Niederland 1971). The fact that adolescents showed a higher rate of psychosomatic diseases suggested an epigenetic development or pattern of emotions. Emotions that are not differentiated and are poorly verbalized cannot be identified as feelings and are not suitable as signals to one's self. Since much information processing, including the preprocessing of perceptions, impulses, cognition, memory, and recall, depends upon the availability of (subliminal) affect signals, the resulting disturbances are widespread. When affects manifest themselves mostly in their somatic undifferentiated form, the subjects tend to ignore all of their body's and mind's signals of danger, and that ascetic attitude coincides with psychosomatic diseases. Conversely, if they develop a dread of these "expressive" elements of emotions and strive to modify or block them by any possible means, there is a propensity to addictive behavior.

In addition there is a blocking of the capacity for wish fulfillment fantasy. As the mental productions become mundane and chronically dominated, the capacity for fantasy, which is necessary for the formation of neuroses, transferences, and fulfilling life patterns, is severely damaged. There is a lack of empathy with objects and a tendency to treat oneself as a robot. Various authors (Marty et al. 1963; Nemiah and Sifneos 1970a, 1970b; McDougall 1974) have demonstrated that in psychosomatic diseases there is a disturbance in cognition called "operative thinking." Sifneos (1967) has coined the word "alexithymia" for this disturbance. I found this same disturbance in my "survivor" population and in individuals who had problems with addictions (Krystal 1962, 1978a).

Moreover, in my studies of alcoholism and drug dependence I found that many of these patients had a history of severe *infantile* psychic trauma (Krystal 1982b, 1982c). It is understandable that in people who have experienced infantile psychic trauma, strong affects are experienced as heralds of trauma and therefore are dreaded and blocked in every way possible. This arrest of the genetic development of affect stands in contrast to the aftereffects of adult trauma in which there is a regression in affective development. Psychotherapeutic intervention in patients with severe alexithymia may be dangerous in that these patients experience just the physiological components of the emotions instead of the feelings. An exacerbation of their psychosomatic disease may occur instead (Sifneos 1967, 1973). Therefore, our future capacity to treat post-traumatic states depends in part on our capacity to diagnose and treat alexithymia and would facilitate effective therapeutic intervention in the other aftereffects of the traumatic state as well.

Continuation of Emergency Regimes

The tendency to continue hypervigilance (Niederland 1961, 1981; Krystal and Niederland 1968) may include physical anxiety responses such as startle patterns, increased muscular tension, and all those components of anxiety which are sometimes referred to as "sympathetic nervous system overactivity." Once the feeling of security has been destroyed, there is an expectation of states of distress. Thus, the fear of recurrence is now known to be one of the regular aftereffects of disaster (Wolfenstein 1957) and of individual stress (Horowitz 1976; Krupnick and Horowitz 1981).

These chronic anxiety states may manifest themselves entirely in physical symptoms (particularly in the presence of alexithymia), or in terms of chronic worry, insecurity, and the like. Repetitive anxiety and persecutory dreams are part of this problem, as may be certain waking confusional states (Niederland 1961, 1981). Various relaxations and retraining techniques may be helpful in modifying these hyperreactivity states.

Continuation of Cognitive Constriction

The constriction of all of the cognitive functions is manifested in one of two basic patterns: (1) a continuation of a general dullness, obtuseness, lowering of performance in familial and occupational spheres; and (2) a tendency to "freeze" or panic suddenly when under pressure.

Pseudophobia

In these states the patients frequently complain that they are afraid of some specific thing such as uniformed men or the sound of explosions or some other object. These will be found referring to the fear of the past. Some individuals may also be afraid of their own dreams, which represent "reruns" of the traumatic past. They have a tendency to take sleeping pills to suppress their own dreaming rather than to regulate their sleep. The chronic intense anxiety may appear to be a matter of multiple phobias; but one finds that these people are often not able to describe what it is they are afraid of.

Dead to the World Reactions

These are the most devastating aftereffects of psychic trauma and have been best described by Murray (1967). He defined "dead to the world" reactions as a cessation of the orientation of conscious life, or as experiencing one's social world as being dead. Being dead to one's inner world means reaching a state of cessation.

An illustration of a man with a dead to the world reaction is given by Wallant (1962) in the screenplay *The Pawnbroker*. This tragic depletion of one's life's resources, a picture of life in death, has been referred to in the Holocaust literature by many authors under many names, among them a "break in the lifeline," or "loss of personality" (Venzlaff 1963).

A lesser, yet very common manifestation of the residue of survivorship of mass destruction is the sense of the meaning of one's life being limited to being a memorial to those who perished. Where the lost relatives and people have fallen victim to an external enemy, these reactions become reinforced by the need to deal with the residual chronic aggression. Once established, the "monument" or "witness against evil" pattern in survivors' lives becomes reinforced also by providing a means to work off some survivor guilt (Krystal 1981).

The Problem of Aggression

The anger that so often has to be suppressed in the traumatic situation only goes underground and returns as a most permanent challenge to the future adjustment of the subject. Its appearance can be marked as soon as safety is reestablished. For instance, in working with adolescent Holocaust survivors, Sterba (1949) found that when brought to this country and placed in foster homes, they gave vent to constant complaints and unbridled aggressive behavior. Hoppe (1962, 1968) found in his therapeutic work with survivors that many developed "reactive aggression" and "hate addiction." He found that the "aggressive survivor who permanently externalizes a part of his superego is fighting against representatives of the externalized negative conscience. The aggression creates new guilt feelings, especially if the survivor's hate addiction turns against his own family members" (Hoppe 1971, p 179). The aftereffects in witnesses or perpetrators of atrocities appear to be predominantly those of aggression. In some Vietnam veterans the problem of aggression appears to be predominant.

The problem of enormous consequences, which has hitherto escaped adequate attention and exploration, is the capacity to exercise self-caring functions. Because of the exclusive focusing on the oedipal conflict in psychoanalysis, we have overlooked the conflictual nature of the assumption and carrying out of self-caring functions. These include a wide scope of activities from those which secure survival to self-soothing, including self-respect regulation. Many of these functions, such as organizing one's thoughts and the regulation of excitement, are commonly experienced as belonging to one's primal object. Hence we are dealing here with the basic issues of self and object representation formation and with problems resulting from identification with the mothering parent (as opposed to the oedipal identification with the parents in regard to phalic and genital strivings).

My findings have shown that in posttraumatic states there is a worsening (extending the scope) of the inhibitions in regard to self-caring and self-soothing (Krystal 1978b). Thus, these patients may, for instance, not feel free to relax and calm themselves when needed, particularly in order to go to sleep. We also run into great resistance when helping them to manage and verbalize their affects, or while teaching them a relaxation technique. The potential of biofeedback techniques has been greatly limited by this unexpected obstacle. I have found that patients who were in psychoanalytic therapy while receiving biofeedback training experienced great guilt as trying to usurp a function which was reserved for mother and appropriate surrogates (transference objects like the doctor, the clinic, etc.). These patients expected that the punishment for this promethean offense was a "fate worse than death"; i.e., the return of the infantile trauma states (Krystal 1978b).

TREATMENT IMPLICATIONS

Situations in which individuals are deprived of their usual supports and thrown into a state of overwhelming helplessness, or into a frame of mind where they break their taboos, particularly against killing, will produce lasting if not irreversible damages. It is useful to separate the concepts of infantile psychic trauma from the adult catastrophic state, even though they share some similar aftereffects such as alexithymia, anhedonia, diminution of affect tolerance, and inhibition of self-caring capacities. It is essential to understand the details and the dynamics of the traumatic process in order to recognize and identify the relevant aftereffects. Terr (1983) utilized insights such as those described here to demonstrate significant aftereffects in the children of the Chowchilla kidnapping four years later. In contrast, lack of familiarity with post-traumatic sequelae will lead to missed diagnoses and inadequate treatment.

The descriptions and the understanding of the sequelae are but a prologue to our approaches to therapy and, ultimately, prevention. But the study of aftereffects itself is as much hampered by obstacles from within the investigators as survivors. Subjects of the trauma may not be at all inclined to volunteer information nor even to view themselves in terms of the victimization. Niederland and I have repeatedly emphasized the problems related to the conspiracy of silence in post-traumatic states (Krystal and Niederland 1968). This reaction needs to be kept in mind both in mass disasters and in individual family affairs. This has been shown clearly in the work of Lister (1982): In situations of child abuse in the family, the victim may have been ordered to be absolutely silent about what happened and therefore will not volunteer any information. Forced silence and secrecy become a problem in postdisaster states both private and public.

An additional problem is that the surviving victim becomes the subject of projection of a multitude of sins that we would rather forget and, therefore, much of the aggression tends to turn to the victim rather than the perpetrator in the postdisaster era. The ambivalence toward the damaged population (veterans, victims of disaster, survivors, and the like) is frequently manifest by a capricious and inconsistent administration of restitution and re-habilitation programs. As an illustration, I found in a study of 367 consecutive cases of survivors of the Nazi Holocaust that there was no correlation between pension or restitution and diagnosis of degree of damage or extent of suffering of the survivors (Krystal 1968a). Restitution determinations were made by bureaucrats who had set up their own policies and procedures, which reflected the orientation of a particular branch of the restitution authorities. To counteract such forces in public policy we must have hard facts about human damage and rehabilitation.

Hoppe (1971) studied the special reactions of psychiatrists when confronting survivors of the persecution. He pointed out the impact upon the therapist in dealing with very painful material— the kind that tends to revive sadomasochistic conflicts within the therapist. Eissler (1967) highlighted the dilemma of intense emotional reactions toward the defeated and humiliated survivor.

The archaic contempt, scorn, or spite for the suffered is rather complex. It is connected with the whole problem of sadomasochism and the reaction to various shades of narcissism. The awe and respect that strongly narcissistic personalities evoke are well known.

The persecuted one, however, has presented a configuration of exactly the opposite character. He has been utterly depleted of any narcissistic cathexis. During his persecution nothing belonged to him any longer—not even his own body. No decision was left to him; he was reduced to sheer nothingness—a state to which not even flattery or civility could be used as a technique of survival. I am compelled to draw the conclusion that among the many causes for hostility towards the victims of persecution, regression to the pagan feeling of contempt for those who are suffering physically must be included. It may well be the most insidious and most potent cause of all. Why some act out that contempt while others are capable of repressing it I do not know. But my belief is that with few exceptions feelings of contempt for suffering are something of a universal reaction still very much alive in almost all of us. (p 1358)

The difficulties in trying to treat such patients with methods and the conceptual tool developed for neurotic patients are obvious. When dealing with individuals who have lived in a psychotic environment and whose reality was beyond the scope of the ordinary life and expectable environment, the therapist must be prepared to deal with extraordinary events, extraordinary ideas, and extraordinary feelings and responses on his or her own part.

References

Allerton CW: Mass casualty care and human behavior. Med Ann Dist Columbia 33:206, 1964

Archibald HC, Long DM, Miller C, et al: Gross stress reaction in combat—a 15 year follow up. Am J Psychiatry 119:317–322, 1962

Bartemeir LH, Kubie LS, Menninger KA, et al: Combat exhaustion. J Nerv Ment Dis 104:358–389, 1946

Bastiaans J: Psychosomatische Gevolgen van onderdrukking en verzet. Amsterdam, North-Holland, 1957

Beebe GW, Appel JW: Variations in Psychological Tolerance to Ground Combat in World War II. Washington, DC, National Academy of Sciences, National Research Council, 1958

Brill NW, Beebe GW: A follow-up study of war neurosis. Veterans Administration Medical Monograph, 1955

Caplan G: Mastery of stress: psychosocial aspects. Am J Psychiatry 128:413–420, 1981

Cohen BM, Cooper MZ: A Follow-up Study of World War II Prisoners of War. Washington, DC, U.S. Government Printing Office, 1954

Dill DB: Human reactions in disaster situation. DN-18-108-CML-2275, National Opinion Research Center. Chicago, University of Chicago, 1954

Eissler KR: Perverted psychiatry? Am J Psychiatry 123:1352–1358, 1967

Erikson KT: Everything in its Path—Destruction of Community in the Buffalo Creek Flood. New York, Simon & Schuster, 1976

Freud S: Introduction to psychoanalysis and the war neuroses (1919), in Complete Psychological Works, standard ed, vol 17. Translated and edited by Strachey J. London, Hogarth Press, 1959

Freud S: Sketches for the "preliminary communication" (1893a), in Complete Psychological Works, standard ed, vol 1. Translated and edited by Strachey J. London, Hogarth Press, 1959

Freud S: Studies on hysteria (1893b), in Complete Psychological Works, standard ed, vol 2. Translated and edited by Strachey J. London, Hogarth Press, 1959

Furst S: Psychic Trauma. New York, Basic Books, 1967

Grinker RR, Spiegel JP: Men Under Stress. New York, Blackiston, 1945

Hoppe KD: Persecution, depression and aggression. Bull Menninger Clin 26:195–203, 1962

Hoppe KD: Psychotherapy with concentration camp survivors, in Massive Psychic Trauma. Edited by Krystal H. New York, International Universities Press, 1968

Hoppe KD: The aftermath of Nazi persecution reflected in recent psychiatric literature, in Psychic Traumatization. Edited by Krystal H, Niederland WG. Boston, Little, Brown, 1971

Horowitz MJ: Stress Response Syndromes. New York, Jason Aronson, 1976

Johnson DA: An experimental evaluation of behavioral inaction under stress. IRAD Technical Report #D23-70-215, McDonnell Douglas Corp Report #g1008, 1970

Kardiner A: The Traumatic Neurosis of War. New York, Basic Books, 1941

Klein M: Notes on some schizoid mechanisms. Int J Psychoanal 27:99–110, 1946

Krupnick JL, Horowitz MJ: Stress response syndromes: recurrent themes. Arch Gen Psychiatry 38:428–435, 1981

Krystal H: The opiate withdrawal syndrome as a state of stress. Psychiatr Q 36:4–65, 1962

Krystal H: Psychotherapy with survivors of Nazi persecution, in Massive Psychic Trauma. Edited by Krystal H. New York, International Universities Press, 1968a

Krystal H: Review of findings and implications of this symposium, in Psychic Traumatization. Edited by Krystal H, Niederland WG. Boston, Little, Brown, 1968b, pp 217–230

Krystal H: Study of juvenile survivors of concentration camps. Unpublished report to discussion group of "Children of Disaster," 1968c

Krystal H: Trauma and the stimulus barrier. Unpublished paper presented at the Annual Meeting of the American Psychoanalytical Association, San Francisco, May 8, 1970

Krystal H: Affect tolerance. Annual of Psychoanalysis 2:179–219, 1974

Krystal H: Psychic trauma and psychogenic death, in Psychiatric Problems in Medical Practice. Edited by Balis GU, Wurmser L, McDaniel E, et al. Boston, Butterworths, 1978a

Krystal H: Trauma and affects, in Psychoanalytic Study of the Child. Edited by Solnit A. New Haven, Yale University Press, 1978b

Krystal H: Integration and self healing in posttraumatic states. J Geriatr Psychiatry 14:165–189, 1981

Krystal H: The activating aspects of emotion. Psychoanal and Contemporary Thought 5:605–642, 1982a

Krystal H: Adolescence and the tendencies to develop substance dependence. Psychoanal Inquiry 2:581–617, 1982b

Krystal H: Character disorders, in Encyclopedic Handbook of Alcoholism. Edited by Pattison EM, Kaufman E. New York, Gardner Press, 1982c

Krystal H, Moore RA, Dorsey JM: Alcoholism and the force of education. Personnel and Guidance Journal 45:134–139, 1966

Krystal H, Moore RA, Dorsey JM: Alexithymia and the effectiveness of psychoanalytic treatment. Int J Psychoanal Psychother 9:353–388, 1982

Krystal H, Niederland WG: Clinical observations on the survivor syndrome, in Massive Psychic Trauma. Edited by Krystal H. New York, International Universities Press, 1968

Krystal H, Niederland WG (eds): Psychic Traumatization. Boston, Little, Brown, 1971

Lifton RJ: Death in Life: Survivors of Hiroshima. New York, Random House, 1968

Lister ED: Forced silence: a neglected dimension of trauma. Am J Psychiatry 139:872–876, 1982

Marty P, de M'Uzan M, David C: L'investigation psychosomatique. Paris, Presses Universitaires, 1963

McDougall J: The psychosoma and the psychoanalytic process. Int Rev Psychoanal 1:437–459, 1974

Minkowski E: L'anesthesie affective. Ann Med Psychol (Paris) 104:8–13, 1946

Murray HA: Dead to the world: passions of Herman Melville, in Essays in Self Destruction. Edited by Shneidman ES. New York, Science House, 1967

Nemiah JC, Sifneos PE: Affect and fantasy in patients with psychosomatic disorders, in Modern Trends in Psychosomatic Medicine. Edited by Hill OW. London, Butterworths, 1970a

Nemiah JC, Sifneos PE: Psychosomatic illness: a problem of communication. Psychother Psychosom 18:154–160, 1970b

Niederland WG: The problem of the survivor. J Hillside Hosp 10:233–247, 1961

Niederland WG: Clinical observations on the "survivor syndrome." Int J Psychoanal 4:313–315, 1968

Niederland WG: Survivor syndrome: further observations and dimensions. J Am Psychoanal Assoc 29:413–416, 1981

Papousek H, Papousek M: Cognitive aspects of preverbal secret interaction, in Parent-Infant Interaction. New York, Associated Science Publishers, 1975

Richter CP: On the phenomenon of sudden death in animals and man. Psychosom Med 19:191–198, 1957

Schur M: Comments on the metapsychology of somatization. Psychoanal Study Child 10:119–164, 1955

Seligman MEP: Helplessness: On Depression, Development and Death. San Francisco, Freeman and Co., 1975

Sifneos PE: Clinical observations on some patients suffering from a variety of psychosomatic diseases, in Proceedings of the Seventh European Conference on Psychosomatic Research. Basel, Karger, 1967

Sifneos PE: The prevalence of "alexithymic" characteristics in psychosomatic patients. Psychother Psychosom 22:257–262, 1973

Snyder SH: Brain peptides as neurotransmitters. Science 209:976–983, 1980

Sterba E: Emotional problems in displaced children. Journal of Casework 30:175–181, 1949

Stern MM: Fear of death and neurosis. J Psychoanal Assoc 16:3–31, 1968a

Stern MM: Fear of death and trauma. Int J Psychoanal 9:458–461, 1968b

Terr L: Chowchilla revisited: the effects of psychic trauma four years after a school bus kidnapping. Am J Psychiatry 140:1543–1550, 1983

Tyhurst JS: Individual reactions to community disasters. Am J Psychiatry 107:764–769, 1951

Venzlaff U: Erlebnifhintergrund und dynamik seelischer verfolgungschaeden, in Psychische Spaetscheden nach politischer Verfolgung. Basel, Karger, 1963

Wallant EC: The Pawnbroker (Screenplay). New York, McFadden, 1962

Wolfenstein M: Disaster: A Psychological Essay. New York, Arno Press, 1957

Zetzel ER: Anxiety and the capacity to bear it. Int J Psychoanal 30:1–12, 1949

Zetzel ER: The incapacity to bear depression (1955), in Capacity for Emotional Growth. New York, International Universities Press, 1970

2

Clinical Implications of the Rorschach in Post-Traumatic Stress Disorder

Bessel A. van der Kolk, M.D.
Charles Ducey, Ph.D.

2

Clinical Implications of the Rorschach in Post-Traumatic Stress Disorder

With the reemergence of an interest in the consequences of psychological trauma there is a rediscovery of the degree to which both the physical and mental states connected with traumatic events continue to be the principal preoccupation in the life of sufferers of post-traumatic stress disorder (PTSD). Kardiner (1941), who first described the full syndrome of PTSD on the basis of his observations of World War I (WWI) veterans, pointed out that sufferers of chronic PTSD continue to live in the emotional environment of the traumatic event, with a continuing perceptual heightening of stimuli signaling threat. Both he and Krystal (1978) observed that people who have been exposed to catastrophic events react to them with the establishment of a new style of adaptation which centers around a restriction of affective involvement with their environment. Thus, while their autonomic nervous system continues to react to some physical and emotional stimuli as if there were a continuing threat of annihilation, they appear to compensate for this hyperreactivity with emotional withdrawal. This withdrawal may have many gradations, ranging from a vague sense of emotional unavailability to an intellectual and emotional deterioration that is not unlike that observed in chronic schizophrenics.

The lives of people with PTSD appear organized around dealing with the aftermath of the trauma: they are either dominated by recurrent intrusive events related to the trauma, in the form of nightmares and flashbacks, or by avoidance of affective involvement lest feelings related to the trauma are reexperienced. However, as Kardiner has pointed out, some parts of the organism are not susceptible to chronic inhibition. The autonomic nervous system continues to prepare the organism for action, but instead of promoting eagerness and curiosity, this activation leads to anxiety, irritability, hyperacusis, and preparedness for flight.

During times of pronounced autonomic activation, either behavioral disturbances or intolerable intrusive traumatic memories will allow for a ready diagnosis of post-traumatic stress disorder. However, when controls predominate and intrusive events are warded off, emotional constriction, chronic passivity, and a vague sense of victimization may be the only apparent sequelae of the trauma, usually missed by the diagnostician who is not alert to the possibility. Among people who fall in the latter category, the diagnosis of PTSD cannot be made with any degree of certainty, until intrusive phenomena start recurring. This is often the case in older veterans around retirement age, in whom nightmares about traumatic events in World War II (WWII) resume when they are faced with the loss of the structure and purpose that their jobs provided. In one survey, about half of WWII combat veterans who were around retirement age had a recurrence of intrusive recollections or nightmares (van der Kolk et al. 1981). On rare occasions, evidence of continuing preoccupation with the trauma may be absent from a patient's conscious mental life and yet be manifested on psychological testing, particularly the Rorschach.

RORSCHACH DATA

Our study of the Roschach in PTSD was part of an effort to study the nature of post-traumatic nightmares (van der Kolk et al. 1984). We did an in-depth psychological study of Vietnam veterans with weekly traumatic nightmares. The average time since discharge from the service was 13 years. All men had the third edition of the *Diagnostic and Statistical Manual of Mental Disorders* (DSM-III)

(American Psychiatric Press 1980) Axis I diagnosis of PTSD, and no other Axis I or Axis II diagnoses, except for alcohol abuse and/or dysthymic disorder, which were thought to be secondary to PTSD by an independent diagnostician. The lack of other DSM-III diagnoses may make this group an unrepresentative sample of Vietnam veterans in the Veterans Administration (VA) system in terms of mental health. All subjects were employed and married. These 15 men were selected for the intensity of their recurrent, intrusive nightmares.

The Roschach protocols of these 15 men fall into two general categories of experience type (Rorschach 1921). There were ten extratensive and three coarctated records, in addition to two unclassified, mixed ones. The markedly extratensive protocols were characterized by (1) extensive, unstructured use of color, not balanced by such ego control functions as are embodied in human movement responses; (2) extensive blood and anatomy content; and (3) uncensored and uncontrolled references to traumatic Vietnam experiences. These records show a high number of color-form (CF) responses (use of color with little structure), a fairly high number of inanimate movement responses (suggesting an intrusive, ego-alien fantasy style [Rorschach 1921]), and a striking absence of W^{++} and W^{+} (well integrated) responses. Human movement responses, thought to indicate a capacity for thinking, fantasy, and planning, were virtually absent from these protocols (Exner 1974).

Color cards (II, III, VIII, IX, X) particularly provoked traumatic response. Table 1 shows representative responses to cards II and VIII by three consecutive subjects in the study. All three subjects were employed (policeman, minister, lawyer) and married and had no clinical evidence of psychosis.

The three coarctated protocols showed (1) very few responses; (2) no responses to color; and (3) little or no human movement responses. Two blind Rorschach raters interpreted these Rorschachs as reflecting rigidly defensive, denying, or repressing personalities. The degree of coarctation reflects, on the one hand, an absence of the use of imagination for planning and thinking as "experimental action" (Freud 1911) and, on the other hand, a lack

Table 1 Subjects' descriptions of Rorschach color cards II and VIII

	RESPONSES TO CARD II	
Subject 1 (L)	Subject 2 (D)	Subject 3 (H)
Phantom, F₄ plane blood (tears up), blood and mud smeared together, pink in the mud, dead dogs, all bloody.	First thing that comes to mind is blood, redness and splotches. Looks like a burn. The clothing and flesh is dark and charred. Blood, as before, in the middle is charred clothing and flesh. Ragged edges like a wound.	What is left of a gook's head after you crank a few rounds into it. Part of skull, blood and blood splattering about. Front of skull coming off. Round comes in and shatters everything. Blood and redness.

	RESPONSES TO CARD VIII	
Subject 1	Subject 2	Subject 3
Rats, blood and urine. You piss on dead gooks. Khesanh was infested with rats. They had a field day eating all the dead bodies. Green areas in a rice paddy.	Pelvis, anatomy vertebrae. Two rats.	Like little lights of cigarette. Gangrenous wound, green, yellow watery around it, like five different objects trying to back away from each other, or holding on to each other, fighting for survival.

of affective responsiveness to the environment and an absence of the use of affect as a signal that permits modulated response. In other words, coarctation indicated a breakdown of the capacity for active coping (Schachtel 1966). The extratensive and coarctated Rorschach records are mirror images of each other; they suggest the failure of active ego adaptation, one in the direction of overwhelmed undercontrol, the other of rigid overcontrol.

The blind raters interpreted these Rorschachs as evidence of the PTSD subjects' inability to integrate immediate affective experience and cognitive structuring of experience. Such lack of integration results in an extreme reactivity to the environment without intervening reflectiveness. The subjects were seen as being aware of tendencies toward uncontrolled and diffuse emotional tension, but unable to articulate specific and differentiated emotions. Most strikingly, these men lack the internal processing mechanisms that might lead to the resolution or integration of trauma. They are unable to differentiate specific affects and to integrate them through introspection and fantasy. Affect is therefore dealt with through unreflective and impulsive action. Hence, though overwhelmed by diffuse affective stimulation, they remain unaware of what they are feeling in specific and differentiated ways.

Typical psychological interpretations of individual protocols included statements such as "the continuity of existence is lost— he can't link up current experiences with the past"; "he is too aware of the fragility of the human body to get involved with intimate attachments"; and "he sees only wounds where others see people"; "he regulates his affect by withdrawal, in the form of figurines, masks, and rejections of individual cards"; "he can't delay action through the use of fantasy"; and "his affect is too overwhelming to make sense of his past experience"; "fear of unbearable affects interfere with accurate form perceptions"; and so on. Some of the PTSD subjects also had markedly elevated scores on Johnston and Holzman's (1979) thought disorder index despite the absence of psychotic thinking on intensive clinical interviews, both structured and unstructured. Hence, overwhelming affective stimuli also led to a disorganization of thought processes.

CASE HISTORY

A specific case example will provide a longitudinal overview of the intimate relationship between a coarctated Rorschach record and denial of affect on the one hand, and an extratensive record and overwhelming affect, on the other. Mr. D came to our clinic in 1972, three years after honorable discharge from the marines. He wanted to be a policeman, and was presently attending community college. His chief complaint was a virtually unremitting headache, occurring "all the time," and reaching debilitating intensity about once a month. He had tried several medicines without relief. He denied excessive use of alcohol and marijuana. The headaches had begun in Vietnam at Thanksgiving, 1968, when he was hit by schrapnel under his right eye and was thrown against a tree, hitting his head and back. Two months after the injury he had "freaked out" on alcohol and marijuana: he had felt paranoid and withdrawn from others, and had broken into sweats and screamed in his sleep. He finished his tour of duty, and had recently been married. His wife told him that he cries in his sleep, and once in his sleep he had punched his wife and had sworn at her. He does not remember these episodes, and states that if he has nightmares he does not remember them.

Mr. D was described by his psychiatrist as very defensive, inappropriately humorous, rather vague about his headaches, and appearing to lack the amount of pain he described. Electroencephalogram (EEG), skull and chest films were normal. The neurologist was unable to conclude that his headaches were specifically related to his head injury. On psychological testing Mr. D's measured intellectual functioning was in the average range. On the Rorschach he only gave ten responses, an unusually low number; he rejected two cards altogether. In the intellectual and the projective tests the examiner felt that Mr. D had difficulty retaining information, integrating thoughts, maintaining a concept, and forming abstractions—in sum, that he was suffering from "mild to moderate brain impairment." The Rorschach protocol's constriction was taken as further evidence of brain damage, and the Rorschach interpretation concluded with the statement that "this protocol shows no evidence of emotional interference, either of an acute or chronic nature."

In October 1975, Mr. D came back to the clinic. He continued to complain of headaches, which were now especially painful in the right temporal area. In 1973 he had had two lumbar disks removed, and he now complained of leg pain. He had been a policeman since 1974, and he had made an apparently good social and marital adjustment.

On New Year's Eve, 1980, Mr. D presented himself at the clinic complaining of flashbacks and hallucinations. He had not slept for five days and was given Dalmane and Serax. On his return appointment two days later he complained of nightmares occurring every night between 2:00 and 3:00 A.M., hypnagogic hallucinations, daytime flashbacks, and startle reactions. In the nightmares and flashbacks he often saw the face of his buddy Bill, whose head was blown off in Vietnam on April 22, 1968, while he was sitting next to Mr. D. Mr. D also had thoughts of committing suicide, and felt constantly anxious and only tenuously in control over violent impulses. On December 20, 1980, he had had a car accident. His automobile was totally destroyed, and he thought he had run over a dog, though he could not find the animal after the wreck.

Mr. D dated the onset of his symptoms to an incident a few months before, in which a man had pulled a knife on him during a robbery. Since this episode he had had nightmares of the incident and of an incident two years earlier in which an emotionally disturbed girl had pulled a knife on him and killed herself.

But mainly, the nightmares pictured his traumatic experiences in Vietnam. During this evaluation Mr. D revealed that he had had traumatic nightmares after returning from Vietnam, but that his year of college and his many friends had helped him to recover. The nightmares, in so far as he remembered them while awake, had ceased until their recent recrudescence.

Two facts about Mr. D's life at the time of the third evaluation are worth noting. First, he had been separated from his wife, who had become pregnant and had an abortion, and now was going blind from diabetes. He had acquired a girlfriend, with whom he was often angry—so angry that he felt like punching her, but he had kicked a hole in the wall instead. Second, he no longer complained of headaches, merely mentioning to the examiner that he used to have very serious ones.

The Rorschach administered to Mr. D during the first evaluation in 1973, when he had repressed his Vietnam experience, differed dramatically from his 1981 Rorschach, administered during his third evaluation, when he presented a fully evident post-traumatic stress disorder. For instance, his bland response to card I in 1973 was "A bat, sort of like the head, the wings spread, and the body. More like a bat than anything else." In 1981, after having seen his life being threatened, and after leaving his terminally ill wife (about whom he denied any feelings), the repression suddenly failed; when presented with the unstructured stimuli of the Rorschach, he slowly and painfully revealed the story of what happened in Vietnam that had never become clear even in lengthy clinical interviews. Card I: "Looks like a Vietnamese whose head I blew off. He had no head. His head blows off from the top of his eyes. Also looks like a bat, also like Jesus Christ nailed to the cross—blotches of blood—the way it is splattered heavy in some areas, lighter in others. Like a pool of blood when you slice somebody open. Also a robe, the robe I see is blood. Yes, maybe clothes covered with the blood of my buddies."

In 1981, on Card II, which he had rejected in 1973, he saw "A woman having a baby. Opening of vagina and blood and everything. Afterbirth. Pulling baby out (he later told he had both raped women and delivered a baby in Vietnam). Two figures in ski masks robbing a store. The opening is myself shrinking away. My head gets to a point where I get scared. The head gets smaller to the size of a nickel. I'd hallucinate walking through mine fields and blowing myself up. I carried a Vietnamese head around after my friend Bill was killed. I cut the head off at the shoulders. The head just shrank. I'm not going to jail like Calley did."

In 1981, Card V: "A monarch butterfly. Actually, it all looks like blood to me. A nice big ton of blood. I see a face in here. I see by buddy Bill who was killed. I killed two Vietnamese because he was killed. I charged into the lines, felt so great that I came in my pants. Then I went back and saw his head blown to bits. I walked around with part of his body, an eye, for a couple of months. I also walked around with a Vietnamese head in my pack until I was medivaced for malaria. I never really believed he was dead. I always expected him on the next transport, but he never did come back. I think I saw Bill's face, without eyes."

In 1981, on Card VI, which he had rejected on the 1973 Rorschach, he saw "One of my buddies cut in half. The Vietnamese like to cut people in half from head to toe. They cut off balls, and stuff them in your mouth and cut you in half. I went crazy. I charged a whole platoon of North Vietnamese. One guy sent a picture to his mother.

The first time I took this test it was a joke. Now I get upset looking at them. I feel like crying. When I said it looked like Bill, it was war. Now I start to stutter when I get angry with people. I black out, I don't know what to say. I feel out of control."

Cards VII, VIII, IX, and, X elicited a continuation of similar responses.

DISCUSSION

These Rorschach responses clearly demonstrate how the trauma and its concomitant affects persist with little modification over time. Repression of the trauma and its recurrence in unmitigated form was the subject of intense scrutiny around the turn of the century. Janet, in his book *The Mental State of Hystericals* (1911), dealt with it in detail:

> Pain is often reexperienced at later points in time much the same manner as in the actual earlier traumatic insult. The trauma remains isolated, more or less completely separated from the other ideas; it can develop and suppress all else. . . .

The concept of psychic trauma was central to Freud's model of mental functioning. After initially formulating a traumatic theory of neurosis (Origins of Psychoanalysis), he gradually abandoned this theory in favor of a more intrapsychic model which emphasized the role of oedipal fantasy in the genesis of neurosis. In this context he developed an elaborate theory of the internal mechanism of repression as the intrapsychic counterpart to the behavioral response of flight from dangerous or painful external stimulation (Freud 1915). After minimizing the impact of actual externally induced trauma for many years, WWI and its aftermath served as a reminder of the role of trauma as a causative principle in neurosis. In "Beyond the Pleasure Principle" (1920) Freud introduced the concept of the stimulus barrier, and its failure to screen out overwhelming excitation in the face of massive psychic trauma:

> The concept of trauma necessarily implies . . . a breach in an otherwise efficacious barrier against stimuli. Such an event as an external trauma is bound to provoke a disturbance on a large scale in the

functioning of an organism's energy and to set in motion every possible defensive measure . . . An "anticathexis" on a grand scale is set up, for whose benefit all the other psychical systems are impoverished, so that the remaining psychical functions are extensively paralysed or reduced. (Freud 1920)

Thus both Janet and Freud were aware of the clinical issues which the Rorschachs in this study demonstrate: the rigidity of defense against trauma, the return of the affective impact of the trauma in its initial and uncontrolled form, and the impoverishment of all other aspects of life when one is absorbed in warding off the impact of the traumatic experience.

People with post-traumatic stress disorder can respond to nonaffective stimuli in a rote manner, but when presented with ambiguous or affectively charged stimuli they respond to current situations as if they were a recurrence of the traumatic stress. Their Rorschachs confirm the clinical impression that people with PTSD are incapable of modulated affective experience; they either respond to affective stimulation with an intensity which is appropriate to the traumatic situation, or they barely react at all. These Rorschachs demonstrate the immediacy of their experience and the lack of capacity to symbolize, fantasize, or sublimate. They appear to be incapable of using fantasy to anticipate or modify emotional responses. Hence, they are deprived of precisely those psychological mechanisms which allow people to cope with the narcissistic injuries of daily life. Our work on traumatic nightmares (van der Kolk et al. 1984) has demonstrated a parallel, concrete, unmodified reliving of the trauma in dreams. Being unable to process affective stimulation through these channels, very few psychological options remain open. Because these patients react to emotional stimulation as a recurrence of the traumatic stress, they respond to any affectively charged situation only through the rigid, primitive, and totalistic reactions appropriate to overwhelming and traumatizing situations—either with fight responses or with flight. This lack of affect tolerance interferes with the ability to grieve, and with the capacity to work through ordinary everyday conflicts and to accumulate restitutive, gratifying experiences.

Emotional constriction is probably the more common form of PTSD, and the diagnosis is usually missed during this phase, as it was in our subject. Mr D's first Rorschach protocol clearly illustrates the price he paid for the withdrawal: emotional barrenness and a life devoid of the adaptive use of fantasy, which prevented a sense of free emotional access to and communication between past, present, and future, with nothing (besides the trauma) to recall and with nothing to look forward to. It is ironic that his doctors thought that he had lost part of his brain.

With the breakthrough of traumatic memories there also is a return of affectivity. There is a fuller range of psychic activity, including fantasy, and there are some whimsical responses among the horror and dysphoria. People return into the picture, even if initially they are only the dead people lost in battle. Our clinical impressions confirm Horowitz's (1973) thesis that integration of the trauma can only occur during the phase of emotional undercontrol.

TREATMENT IMPLICATIONS

Krystal (1978) has pointed out that the learning of affect tolerance is the first priority in psychotherapy. This may sometimes need to be supplemented by medications that decrease the level of autonomic activation (van der Kolk 1983). Exploration of the nature of the traumatic experience is essential for patients to learn to distinguish between past and present threats. Only after understanding is gained about the totality and meaning of the traumatic event and its delimited place in the person's life can an affective link with both pre-traumatic and post-traumatic people and events be established. Therefore, one needs to trace back the current intense affectivity to the appropriate past stimulus with the expectation that, over time, current life events can be less colored by the affects belonging to traumatic events. Horowitz (1973) has demonstrated the need to understand the character defenses which a person brings to coping with catastrophic trauma in order to overcome resistances and allow a working through.

Given the fact that the central psychological preoccupation in these people's lives is either the reliving or the warding off of the memory of the trauma, there is little room for new, gratifying experiences which might allow for reparation of past narcissistic injuries. Only after the patient is capable of separating the affects belonging to past events from those appropriate to current experiences will he be able to regain a sense of personal history with a past, a present, and a future.

References

American Psychiatric Association: Diagnostic and Statistical Manual of Mental Disorders, 3rd ed. Washington, DC, American Psychiatric Association, 1980

Exner J Jr: The Rorschach: A Comprehensive System, vols 1 & 2. New York, John Wiley & Sons, 1974

Freud S: Formulations on the two principles of mental functioning (1911), in Complete Psychological Works, standard ed, vol 12. Translated and edited by Strachey J. London, Hogarth Press, 1959

Freud S: Repression (1915), in Complete Psychological Works, standard ed, vol 14. Translated and edited by Strachey J. London, Hogarth Press, 1959, pp 141-158

Freud S: Beyond the Pleasure Principle (1920), in Complete Psychological Works, standard ed, vol 18. Translated and edited by Strachey J. London, Hogarth Press, 1959

Horowitz MJ: Phase oriented treatment of stress response syndromes. Am J Psychother 27:506-515, 1973

Janet P: The Mental State of Hystericals. Paris, Alcan, 1911

Johnston MH, Holzman PS: Assessing Schizophrenic Thinking. San Francisco, Jossey-Bass, 1979

Kardiner A: The Traumatic Neuroses of War. New York, Hoeber, 1941

Krystal H: Trauma and affects. Psychoanal Study Child 33:81-116, 1978

Rorschach H: Psychodiagnostik. Bern, Hans Huber Verlag, 1921

Schachtel E: Experiential Foundations of Rorschach's Test. New York, Basic Books, 1966, p 186

van der Kolk, BA: Psychopharmacological issues in the treatment of post-traumatic stress disorder. Hosp Community Psychiatry 34:683–691, 1983

van der Kolk BA, Burr WA, Blitz R, et al: Characteristics of nightmares among veterans with and without combat experience. Sleep Research 10:179, 1981

van der Kolk BA, Blitz R, Burr WA, et al: Nightmares and trauma. Am J Psychiatry 141:187–190, 1984

3

Building a Conceptual Bridge Between Civilian Trauma and War Trauma: Preliminary Psychological Findings from a Clinical Sample of Vietnam Veterans

Jacob D. Lindy, M.D.
Mary C. Grace, M.Ed., M.S.
Bonnie L. Green, Ph.D.

3

Building a Conceptual Bridge Between Civilian Trauma and War Trauma: Preliminary Psychological Findings from a Clinical Sample of Vietnam Veterans

This chapter represents a status report on research in progress at the University of Cincinnati Traumatic Stress Study Center. This group has been studying the psychological effects of disaster on survivors for more than ten years.

Faculty at the center join two lines of investigation. The psychoanalytic/clinical line concerns itself with describing phenomena from a dynamic viewpoint and suggesting what may be effective in outreach to and treatment of survivors. The experimental line operationalizes these descriptions, identifies variables that influence outcome, and measures effectiveness of intervention. Together, the group has developed models that describe the course of posttraumatic stress, predict psychopathology, and assess treatment outcome. Two major research projects studying long-term impairment of survivors of civilian disasters have been completed by the group. In 1972, a dam collapsed at Buffalo Creek, West Virginia, flooding and destroying most of the hamlets beneath it and killing 125 persons (Gleser et al. 1981; Titchener and Kapp 1976). In 1977, a fire destroyed the large Beverly Hills supper club complex near Cincinnati, Ohio. Twenty-five hundred were present at the time; 165 were killed (Green et al. 1983; Lindy et al. 1983).

Members of the Traumatic Stress Study Center have also served in a variety of clinical, consultative, and research capacities in tornadoes, plane crashes, explosions, and other civilian disasters. (These disasters include the Jefferson Grain Explosion [1978], the Algona and Manson, Iowa tornadoes [1979], the Wichita Falls, Texas tornado [1979], the Three Mile Island Nuclear Accident [1979], the Riverfront Coliseum Crash [1979], and the Canadian Airlines Crash [1983].) In those instances where an in-depth investigation is undertaken, our work has included (a) careful narrations of individual survivors' experiences as recorded by trained clinicians, (b) quantification of stressors and symptoms using standardized instruments for both survivor self-reports and interviewer-based data, and (c) treatment and follow-up where possible.

In the process of these investigations, we have elaborated working models for the etiology and natural history of post-traumatic states. Figure 1 is a natural history model. It suggests that factors on three planes—traumatic stressor, personality, and social and environmental support—interplay in complex ways over time in the development and course of post-traumatic stress disorder (PTSD).

We shall first describe briefly a progression through each of the three planes of the model and their interaction over time. Later in the chapter, we shall present data which illustrate individual variability of the contructs under study. Let us first turn to the stressor "plane" of the model.

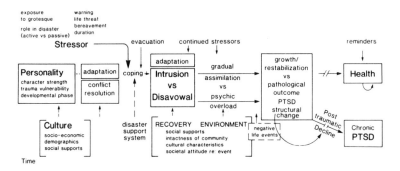

Figure 1 Natural History Model of PTSD and Disaster

Stressors in disaster are not uniform, nor are they limited to a single point in time. Some of the important characteristics of the traumatic stressor are threat to life, bereavement, degree of warning, and exposure to the grotesque. In the aftermath of catastrophe, stressors may be ongoing and new stressors may develop, as in the subsequent disruption in the community at Buffalo Creek (Erikson 1976). Later, even after the event and its aftermath are past, reminders of the stress can recur spontaneously through trigger stimuli (such as rain for Buffalo Creek survivors) and through anniversary reactions. Van der Kolk's excellent case history presented in another chapter of this monograph is an example of "reminders" acting as long-term stressors in the psychopathology of PTSD.

We begin the personality plane of our model with an assessment of premorbid personality factors, such as vulnerability to trauma on the basis of early childhood experiences, developmental phase, and character strength. The personality is thus equipped with a given capacity to adapt to external stress and to resolve internal conflict. When trauma intensity is manageable and personality resources sufficient, the trauma is worked through in a dosed manner, and the stress reaction will be limited. When these resources are inadequate or continually being overwhelmed by intense recurrent intrusive images, the survivor experiences chronic psychic overload and PTSD develops. The intrusion-denial cycle forwarded by Horowitz (1976) is central to this model. Intrusions during sleep may be seen as nightmare/night terror syndrome (see Chapter 5). The personality's long-term efforts to cope under conditions of continuing psychic overload produce secondary character change (Lindy and Titchener 1983). Chronic efforts to ward off recurrence of the trauma produce or reinforce traits such as hypervigilence, alienation, and explosiveness. Efforts to manage intrusive symptoms by self-medication (with alcohol or drugs) introduces further complexity into the clinical picture. Together these changes precipitate a downward spiral of negative life events such as divorce, job loss, legal difficulties. The final clinical picture is described as post-traumatic decline (Titchener and Kapp 1978).

Similarly, constructs along the sociocultural plane of the model are neither unidimensional nor confined to a single point in time. In a general way, cultural background tends to define a survivor's approach to disaster be it a Texan's grand optimism (as in the tornado at Wichita Falls) or an Appalachian withdrawal into the familial (as at Buffalo Creek). Social support in the immediate preparation for disaster can vary widely, as in the premature reassurances at Three Mile Island which threatened lives and engendered profound mistrust, as opposed to the effective media information which saved lives at Wichita Falls. In the early aftermath, survivors may return to intact homes and communities (as in the supper club fire) or their social fabric may have been destroyed through the dislocations following disaster as at Buffalo Creek. The communities that survivors reenter may share in communal mourning or they may turn against the survivor as if he or she were to blame for the catastrophe, as with the Vietnam veteran.

In 1980 our group began building a bridge between the work in civilian disaster and that following war trauma by turning our attention to combatant survivors of the Vietnam War. In the following discussion, we shall present preliminary data from two of our projects with veterans. The first study sample is a group of 26 veterans from a Vietnam Veteran Outreach Center first seen in the summer and fall of 1981. This study was designed initially to develop and test instruments to be used in a larger study. The second study sample is a group of 22 combat veterans referred after April 1982 for individual psychotherapy. This latter study aims primarily at examining treatment outcome. (Both the outreach and the treatment samples are conceptualized as clinical.) In addition, a third study sample consisting of the first 70 subjects in an NIMH project currently underway (intentionally seeking a wider range in current adjustment) will be used. This chapter will address each plane of the disaster and PTSD model: traumatic stressor, personality (its functional impairment and premorbid antecedents), and social supports. We shall use preliminary data from the above samples to clarify a range of research questions in each of these areas.

PSYCHIATRIC IMPAIRMENT

Demographics

Let us now turn to our two clinical samples, beginning with the 26 Vietnam veterans in the outreach study. The sample does not pretend to be representative of Vietnam veterans at large. Rather, it is a volunteer group drawn from veterans in a midwest urban outreach center. While these veterans are not seeking psychotherapy in the traditional sense, they have been drawn to a center which endorses group support to fellow veterans, rap groups, and counseling. It is, therefore, closer to a clinical than a nonclinical group. The mean age is 33; the age at time of combat was 19; and two-thirds are white. Most have now completed high school and half have some additional education. Only 48 percent were employed at the time of the study. Approximately half are married. Distribution among Army, Air Force, Navy, and Marines and years spent in Vietnam is comparable to overall distribution of American forces in Vietnam. The second group, the treatment group, has fewer blacks and more who are currently married than the outreach group. It is otherwise quite similar to the outreach group in basic demographics.

Diagnosis

We now turn to some problems in diagnostic classification of these samples, in particular, problems in differential diagnosis and multiple diagnoses. For purposes of operationalizing diagnosis, we have used the Schedule for Affective Disorders and Schizophrenia-Lifetime (SADS-L). However, at the time that this study began, PTSD was not part of the differential diagnosis assessed by this instrument. It was necessary, therefore, to construct an added section of the SADS-L based in part on the work of Hough and Gongola (1982).

Our next diagnostic problem is that elements of PTSD are commonly seen in other disorders. For example, intrusive images may be difficult to distinguish from hallucinations seen in thought disorder; psychic numbing and/or extreme irritability are seen in mood disorders; and reenactments may appear as acting out behavior seen in personality disorders. Estrangement and alienation are hallmarks of schizotypal disorders, suspiciousness and distrust suggest paranoid disorder, and episodes of explosive behavior suggest borderline personality disorder. This overlap presents a difficulty. Are we describing patients with a single illness (PTSD), who because of diagnostic imprecision and typology overlap, are being recorded as having evidence of other illnesses such as affective disorder or schizotypal, paranoid, or borderline personality disorder. Or are we finding a clinical group with multiple independent diagnoses of which posttraumatic stress disorder is only one (and perhaps a minor one). The following data illustrate the diagnostic dilemma.

In the outreach sample, two-thirds of the patients met criteria for more than one Axis I diagnosis. The third edition of the *Diagnostic and Statistical Manual of Mental Disorders* (DSM-III) (American Psychiatric Association 1980) criteria for post-traumatic stress disorder were met by 71 percent in the outreach sample and 81 percent in the treatment sample. A similar percent met criteria for major affective disorders. Nearly half met criteria for substance abuse (of these, two-thirds were alcohol only). Twenty-seven percent met criteria for anxiety disorders. (These are retrospective diagnoses at any point in time in history of the individual veteran.) Green and others discuss the implications of multiple Axis I diagnoses in more detail in a companion paper (Green BL, Lindy JD, Grace MC: Post-traumatic stress disorder: making the diagnosis and assessing treatment effectiveness. Manuscript submitted for publication).

Personality disorders were assessed with the 128-item Personality Disorder Questionnaire (PDQ) being developed by Hyler and Rieder (1980) of the New York Psychiatric Institute's Biometric Research Lab. These items are true-false statements which the subject answers about himself in the present. Its use in this project is part of field tests for its validity and reliability. Again we have the issue of multiple diagnoses in that nearly half of the outreach subjects meet the criteria for more than one personality disorder.

The common triad in this outreach group was schizotypal (67 percent), paranoid (63 percent), and borderline (67 percent). The PDQ, a self-report instrument, did not pick up antisocial personality disorder in this group to any appreciable degree; however, the SADS-L, an interviewer-based instrument, picked up 23 percent. Frequency of personality disorders in the treatment group was even more striking: schizotypal (100 percent), paranoid (86 percent), borderline (71 percent).

Looking at the total number of pathological responses on the PDQ, (0-128 range), the outreach sample shows a mean of 44.8 while the treatment group is even higher (mean = 53.7). Thus, as a group, this is a clinical population with severe personality trait disturbances. The implications of these findings for preexisting personality disturbances is discussed later.

Levels of Impairment

An ongoing interest of our research group has been the development of a common scientific data base regarding levels of impairment following exposure to differing, massively traumatic experiences. In our previous work, we have elected to utilize Spitzer and Endicott's (1968) Psychiatric Evaluation Form (PEF), a clinical rating (along 19 dimensions) based on a structured interview. The particular advantage of this scale is that it can be scored on the basis of carefully conducted mental status examinations (with impairment being conceptualized as falling along a continuum from none to extreme). Second, we have utilized the 90-item Symptom Checklist (SCL-90) (Derogatis 1977) as a standardized self-report of symptom distress.

Our veteran outreach sample shows an overall or global severity rating of 3.9 (range 1-6 on the PEF)—notably more impaired than the average rating of a large outpatient sample collected by authors of the instrument (3.3). On the SCL-90 also, the outreach group's mean total score of 140.1 (range of 0-360) is higher than scores for patients in an outpatient setting collected by the authors, whereas the treatment group's mean total score of 200 approaches that for inpatient groups.

Table 1   Comparison of Impairment Scores of Vietnam Veterans and Other Clinical Samples

Sample Groups	SCL Total Score (0–360 range)	SCL Hostility Subscale (0–24)
Vietnam Veterans (Outreach)	140.1	10.2
Vietnam Veterans (Treatment)	208.3	—
Buffalo Creek*	79.9 (151)	—
Beverly Hills (Outreach)	57.5	3.5
Beverly Hills (Treatment)	118	7.5
Three Mile Island	43.2	—
Crisis Clinic	132.6	7.5

*Based on 48-item earlier version of SCL; parentheses show converted comparison score.

While the PEF and SCL-90 have the advantage of allowing comparison to other patient samples, they are both general measures of impairment and are not specific for PTSD. A better instrument in this regard is the Impact of Events Scale, which scores symptoms of both intrusion and denial of the traumatic event(s) (Horowitz 1979).

Table 1 compares the level of impairment in the outreach Vietnam veteran group with other clinical and nonclinical survivor samples (namely, the Buffalo Creek Dam Collapse in West Virginia, 1972; the Beverly Hills Supper Club Fire in 1977; the Three Mile Island Nuclear Accident, and a comparison group who are currently seeking treatment in a crisis clinic in our University Hospital.) Self-reports (SCL-90) show our sample as located midway between survivors of the Buffalo Creek Disaster two years after the event and those seeking help at a current crisis clinic. They are more impaired than the clinical sample presenting itself one year following the Supper Club fire. Mothers of young children within five miles of the Three Mile Island area at one year were considerably less symptomatic (Bromet 1981).

TRAUMATIC STRESSORS

In earlier work at Buffalo Creek, there was impressive evidence that two stressors stand out as increasing risk of long-term pathology: threat to life and bereavement (Gleser et al. 1981). These findings were confirmed in studies of the Beverly Hills fire (Green BL, Grace MC, Gleser GC: Identifying survivors at risk: long-term impairment following the Beverly Hills supper club fire. Manuscript submitted for publication). In addition, careful examination of narratives in these studies highlighted additional stressors that were not suspected initially. For example, at Beverly Hills, the handling of dead bodies was identified as an important specific stressor. The task of translating this finding of specificity of stressor to the work with Vietnam veterans is not an easy one.

Unlike civilian disasters, trauma, loss, and exposure to the grotesque were continual for one year. Unlike the passive role of victim in civilian disaster, the combat veteran entered as an agent supposedly prepared for his task. Unlike survivors of the flood or fire, 15 years have now elapsed in the lives of the combat veterans since their tour in Vietnam. Early studies of Vietnam veterans failed to distinguish carefully among the many types of experiences veterans went through while there. More recently, investigators including Boulanger and Smith (1980) and Wilson and Krause (1982) have compiled lists of specific stressors within the Vietnam experience. These fall into two categories: (1) combat role scales in which a dangerous military activity such as carrying out a long-range perimeter patrol is identified; and (2) scales which relate to specific traumatic experiences such as witnessing friends being killed or seeing or participating in body counts or mutilations.

Veterans in the outreach sample participated repeatedly in 7.9 of 23 possible high danger combat roles. In the treatment sample, they participated in 9.4 of 23 possible high danger combat roles. Their scores on frequency of exposure to specific war stressors were outreach 91.5 (26.9) and treatment 102.7 (27.0) (range = 0–180).

Of special interest is the role of certain activities in predicting current functioning. At a preliminary level, our work is consistent with that of Laufer and his group (reported in this monograph) who have identified exposure to abusive violence as having an important effect on later functioning. Over 50 percent of veterans both in the treatment group and the outreach group responded positively to questions dealing with hurting, killing, and mutilating Vietnamese either directly as a participant or indirectly as an observer. Already, process data on therapies have proven particularly interesting as well as instructive in working with a therapeutically difficult patient group. Statistically, the specific stressor variable of exposure to abusive violence will be carefully scrutinized in our final analyses of both the treatment sample and the wide-range study.

PREMORBID FACTORS

A number of confounding problems make examination of the interrelationship between premorbid personality and expression of PTSD and other psychopathology particularly difficult:

1. reliable premorbid data are difficult to obtain;
2. retrospective self-reports may be unreliable;
3. character pathology may have functioned to some extent in Vietnam as a selector both of those who were assigned to dangerous combat conditions and of those who survived;
4. it is possible that some character pathology we see 13 years later may have been secondary to the trauma rather than preceding it;
5. as outlined above, some indicators of character pathology may indeed be overlapping characteristics of PTSD itself.

In the preceding discussion, we grouped personality disorder with other measures of posttrauma pathology. A more conventional view would be to consider current personality disorder as a measure of preexisting personality disturbance. In the latter light, one could infer that our sample was an impaired group prior to Vietnam. However, when we turn to other measures of premorbid functioning such as childhood trauma and adolescent functioning, our preliminary evidence calls into question such unidimensional explanations. One would assume that in lifelong personality disorders, one would find high childhood trauma and poor adolescent functioning. According to these scales, at least some in our clinical groups were indeed well functioning before Vietnam.

The section of the SADS-L related to quality of adolescent friendship was scored independently and correlated with presence of PTSD in the outreach sample. Those who report poor adolescent friendship are less likely to meet clinical criteria for PTSD. Conversely, those who report good adolescent friendships are more likely to meet criteria for PTSD. Our index of childhood vulnerability to trauma employs a modification of a scale developed at the Chicago Psychoanalytic Institute. Preliminary sorting of childhood trauma data yields three groups: (1) no childhood trauma, (2) childhood trauma present but in the presence of a supportive environment, and (3) childhood trauma in the absence of a supportive environment. In the clinical portion of our wide range sample, 33 percent report no childhood trauma, 43 percent present in supportive environment, and 24 percent report trauma in a negative holding environment.

Clinically, we are seeing some patients with apparently good premorbid adjustments, low childhood trauma, and good adolescent relationships who experience prolonged and intense trauma in Vietnam and present with severe PTSD. Just how this breakdown of premorbid factors will ultimately relate to PTSD must await further careful study.

SOCIAL SUPPORTS

At Buffalo Creek, a disruptive and nonfunctional recovery environment was part of the devastation and thought to be clearly related to the high level of impairment found two years later (Erikson 1976). The factor of a rejecting environment at homecoming (Wilson and Kraus 1982; Figley 1980) has been an important theme in the literature on the Vietnam veteran. However, the examination of social support systems in the context of Vietnam is complex. First, there is the immediate social support during this time of a catastrophe; that is, the presence and effectiveness of medical support, the nature of cohesiveness within the combat unit, and the feeling of integrity along the chain of command. Second, there is the extensive period following the war in the American "recovery environment," which often provided a largely negative albeit changing support system. The individual's choice of social networks, both with regard to density and frequency of contact, plays an ongoing role in psychological functioning.

Psychotherapy

The 22 patients in the treatment sample are being seen in once weekly psychotherapy by analysts at the Cincinnati Psychoanalytic Institute for one year. Follow-up measures will be gathered at 18 months in both the treatment group and in the outreach group. Since no publicly funded individual psychotherapy was available to participants in the outreach sample at that time, that group will serve as a naturally occurring comparison group for the treatment study.

The goals of these treatments are to process the veteran's disavowed traumatic experiences in a dosed manner to provide reconstruction of those traumatic experiences in Vietnam which continue to exert excessive influence on current functioning, and to examine the connections between these events and their meaning to precombat and current life. Stepping back from the details of our discussion and appreciating the enormity of the trauma—the 15-year aftermath, the difficulties in establishing social supports, the extent of impairment, the complexity of multiple diagnoses—we are cautioned to be modest in the therapeutic ambition with regard to psychosocial interventions. The goal of successful therapies may be more related to reversing progressive decline, to gaining some sense of personal continuity, and perhaps to regaining integrity and personal meaning, but may well fall short of "cure" in the sense of total symptom removal.

Careful examination of these treated cases should clarify some specific issues in the technique of psychotherapy with chronic PTSD as well as test the efficacy of one particular treatment mode. In addition, we hope that it will also shed light on some ongoing basic research concerns.

1. To what extent is PTSD a primary diagnosis in these cases?
2. If the specific stressors such as abusive violence are particular predictors of long-term pathology, what are the dynamics of such cases and how are they distinguished from other cases of chronic PTSD?
3. Since, in theory, evidence of current personality disorder may be considered as either evidence of premorbid pathology and/or the result of fending off trauma, what changes in indices of personality disorder follow successful focal psychotherapy?

References

American Psychiatric Association: Diagnostic and Statistical Manual of Mental Disorders, 3rd ed. Washington, DC, American Psychiatric Association, 1980

Boulanger G, Smith JR: Traumatic stress reaction scale. 1980

Bromet E, Dunn L: Mental health of mothers nine months after the Three Mile Island accident. Urban and Social Change Review Vol 14, No. 2, 1981

Derogatis LR: SCL-90R Version Manual-I. Baltimore, Johns Hopkins University Press, 1977

Erikson K: Everything in Its Path. New York, Simon and Schuster, 1976

Figley C, Leventman S: Strangers at Home: Vietnam Veterans Since the War. New York, Praeger, 1980

Gleser GC, Green BL, Winget CN: Prolonged Psychosocial Effects of Disaster: A Study of Buffalo Creek. New York, Academic Press, 1981

Green BL, Grace MC, Lindy JD, et al: Levels of functional impairment following a civilian disaster: the Beverly Hills supper club fire. J Consul Clin Psychol 51:573–580, 1983

Horowitz MJ: Stress response syndromes. New York, Jason Aronson, 1976

Horowitz M, Wilner N, Alvarez W: Impact of events scale: a measure of subjective stress. Psychosom Med 41(3):209–218, 1979

Hough R, Gongola P: Post-traumatic stress disorder structured interview. Unpublished study in progress, 1982

Hyler and Reider: Personality disorder questionnaire. Biometrics Research Laboratory, New York State Psychiatric Institute, 1980

Lindy JD, Titchener JL: Acts of God and man: long-term character change in survivors of disasters and the law. Behavioral Sciences and the Law, Vol 3, July 1983

Lindy JD, Green BL, Grace MC, et al: Psychotherapy with survivors of the Beverly Hills supper club fire. Am J Psychother 37:593–610, 1983

Spitzer RL, Endicott J, Mesnikoff AM, et al: The psychiatric evaluation form. New York, Biometrics Research, 1968

Titchener JL, Kapp FT: Family and character change at Buffalo Creek. Am J Psychiatry 133:295–299, 1976

Titchener JL, Kapp FT: Post-traumatic decline. Paper presented at the American Psychoanalytic Association Meeting, New York, 1978

Wilson JP, Krauss GE: Predicting post-traumatic stress syndromes among Vietnam veterans. Paper presented at 25th Neuropsychiatric Institute, VA Medical Center, Coatesville, Pa, October 1982

4

Post-Traumatic Stress Disorder (PTSD) Reconsidered: PTSD Among Vietnam Veterans

Robert S. Laufer, Ph.D.
Elizabeth Brett, Ph.D.
M.S. Gallops, M.Phil.

Post-Traumatic Stress Disorder (PTSD) Reconsidered: PTSD Among Vietnam Veterans

All studies of psychological and behavioral problems among Vietnam veterans use some measure of war stress. The most common dimension of war stress used in these is combat exposure. Although the measures of combat that have been used vary significantly from each other, three combat measures that have been utilized in more than one study (those of Figley 1978; Wilson and Krauss 1980; Harris 1980; and Laufer et al. 1981) have yielded consistent results. The findings generally indicate that combat exposure has a linear relationship with certain current problem outcomes.

Several studies have also shown that there are other dimensions of war stress which are significantly related to long-term disruptive psychosocial patterns (Foy 1981; Wilson and Krauss 1982; Laufer et al. 1984a; Yager et al. in press; Laufer et al. 1983a, 1983b; Laufer and Gallops 1983). The common finding in the Foy (1981) and the Laufer and others studies is that participation in abusive violence plays an important role in long-term adjustment patterns. Foy found that the length of stress exposure, represented by the number of tours of duty, also plays an important role in stress disorder. Wilson and Krauss (1982) and Laufer and others (1984a) have found evidence that subjective responses to stress exposure in war contribute to post-traumatic stress symptomatology; and Wilson and Krauss (1982) found indications of adverse effects as a result of the physical environment, e.g., the terrain and the weather.

The third edition of the *Diagnostic and Statistical Manual of Mental Disorders* (DSM-III) (1980) criterion for the diagnosis of post-traumatic stress disorder (PTSD) requires the specification of a stressor capable of creating "symptoms of distress in almost everyone." This requirement necessitates an approach slightly different from the one in the social psychology of mental health advocated by Wheaton (1983), in which stress is studied by focusing on the manner in which the impact of life events is mediated by the "coping resources and/or the behavioral coping styles of individuals exposed to events." In PTSD research, the investigator must identify the relevant stressors regardless of the coping styles or resources of individuals exposed to the events. There is considerable variability in the nature of stressors across the subareas of the field of stress research. Life event research, for example, deals generally with chronic not traumatic stress. Disaster research, on the other hand, tends to be concerned with short-term traumatic stress. Research on combatants or survivors of war is concerned with both chronic and traumatic stress (Kardiner 1947; Grinker and Spiegel 1945; Krystal and Niederland 1971). With two exceptions (Wilson and Krauss 1982; Laufer et al. 1984a), the literature on post-traumatic stress has not systematically attempted to conceptualize the nature of war stress and formulate a methodological approach to the issue. In this chapter we will discuss the nature of war stress and then examine the relationship between war stress and post-traumatic stress symptomatology and disorder.

War is an example of a class of social trauma where individuals are exposed for extended periods of time to an environment latent with severe stress. One way to conceptualize exposure to extreme stress in these environments is to see them as elements of the individual's "stress career." In Vietnam, soldiers generally served a one year tour of duty, thus each veteran had a "war stress career" of one year, which requires specification.

War stress is a complex phenomenon. There are a number of

questions which must be addressed in any consideration of the nature of war stress. First, we must ask whether or not individual events are to be treated separately or whether the nature of war stress is best understood as a cumulative experience. Second, we must ask whether or not each event ought to be given equal weight or if it is more appropriate to differentiate certain aspects of the war experience into separate categories. Third, while the DSM-III stressor criterion narrows the range of possible stressors so that the individual's coping response is less central, we must specify the relationship between the objective and subjective components of a stressful experience. The answers to these three questions are of paramount importance in understanding how to approach the measurement of war stress.

THE STRESSORS OF WAR

A fundamental issue that must be considered is whether traumatic stress should be treated as particular events which have significant effects on long-term symptomatology or whether we are dealing with sets of stressors which have cumulative effects. The clinical literature has always emphasized the debilitating effects on the soldier of the constant strain inherent in warfare. Grinker and Spiegel (1945) and Kardiner and Spiegel (1947) both state that ordinarily the individual becomes vulnerable to a traumatic neurosis only after prolonged exposure to severe stress, at which point a threshold is reached. The decreased adaptive capacity resulting from cumulative stress is a formal requirement for the development of a traumatic neurosis in Grinker and Spiegel's model. The research literature primarily employs such cumulative measures of stress. The basis of this approach can be found in the early work of Stouffer et al. (1949), who studied the effects of combat on World War II soldiers. Stouffer points out that any individual event may or may not be traumatic in and of itself; the character of specific events or actions that individuals undertake are perceived quite differently by various actors. Nonetheless, the cumulation of a range of activities common to warfare tend to lead to psychiatric problems and psychological responses that are qualitatively distinct and have long-term implications for the mental health of the individual.

This discussion has relevance to a second issue, the need to distinguish classes of traumatic stressors. In the early literature on Vietnam veterans the initial approach to the measurement of traumatic stress was to construct a measure of combat exposure, although some of the very early studies only differentiated between service in Vietnam and service in the military in places other than Vietnam. Measuring combat exposure only is a severely limited approach. Research has consistently shown that there is a range of experiences which is conceptually and empirically distinct from combat, such as exposure to abusive violence (Foy 1981; Wilson and Krauss 1982; Laufer et al. 1984a, 1984b). This recent evidence supports the view that differentiation of classes of war stressors is an essential step in specifying the relationship between traumatic war stress and long-term stress symptomatology and disorder.

While our focus is, in large part, confined to a limited exploration of the war stressors available in our data, we feel it is worth describing the full set of factors which need to be incorporated into a model of war stressors.[1] (Notes appear after the reference list.) This enumeration is tentative, yet it provides a sense of the complexity of the subject and the need for comprehensive examination of the relative significance of these factors in determining long-term stress symptomatology.

Combat

As already indicated, combat is the most commonly used cumulative measure of war stress. The measurement of combat has been as complex an issue as the underlying meaning attributed to the concept has been diverse. In our view, three aspects of combat constitute the essential elements responsible for its effects on veterans over the life course. First, the combat experience should measure the extent to which the individual's life was threatened or at risk. Second, combat involves, at least potentially, the taking of life or inflicting serious injury on others. And third, the combat experience involves the frequency with which the veteran was exposed to life-threatening situations (Figley 1978; Laufer et al. 1981; Foy 1981; Wilson and Krauss 1980). Subsequent studies have all utilized one or more of these aspects of the combat phenomenon in the construction of their measures (Card 1983; Brett 1983; Hough et al. 1983; Polk 1980; Harris 1980).[2]

Exposure to Abusive Violence

Participation in and witnessing abusive violence are two additional measures of war stress found to be important in assessing the effects of the war experience. The stress of war in a guerrilla campaign differs in kind from that experienced in conventional conflicts. Many of the strains placed on conventional forces in a guerrilla campaign stem from the inability of these forces to distinguish between noncombatants and the enemy. This problem is, for the most part, absent in a conventional conflict. Guerrilla warfare creates pressures that lead to and sanction acts of brutality against civilians and prisoners of war. The American experience in Vietnam saw a significant number of such episodes by the North Vietnamese, Vietcong, South Vietnamese, and American forces. In our transcripts from the *Legacies of Vietnam* study, three general types of episodes were described: actions against civilians, actions against prisoners of war (POWs), and the use of cruel weaponry, i.e., abusive violence. In the *Legacies* sample, 22 percent of the Vietnam veterans witnessed abusive violence and 9 percent participated in such actions (Laufer 1984a).[3]

The Death or Wounding of Friends

Considerable evidence exists that the death or serious injury of a friend or someone the veteran was close to in his unit could be a major source of stress in Vietnam. The literature on Vietnam makes this point clearly and unambiguously. There is also evidence that the loss associated with such an event haunts veterans in civilian life. The lasting traumatic effect of such stress is especially evident if the veteran feels, rightly or wrongly, that he could somehow have prevented the death or injury or was responsible for the casualty. Little attention has so far been given to whether or not exposure to this type of trauma functions as an independent stressor.

Isolation from Peers

The rotation system in Vietnam has long been considered an important factor in creating stress in Vietnam veterans because it rotated men singly in and out of units in a tour lasting 365 days (Moskos 1970). Thus, units were composed of men strung out along time lines that were entirely individuated. In each unit were men who were short timers, new guys, and others in the middle months of their tours, familiar with combat and survival techniques. The differences between the times individuals began their tours has given rise to the assertion that in Vietnam it was more difficult than in World War II for soldiers to get close to each other. Closeness created stress because each soldier came to realize he was fundamentally on his own; close attachments involved the hazards of being abandoned as friends left or, alternatively, abandoning friends as the tour ended.

Contact with Death and Dying Outside Combat

A number of activities were common in Vietnam that consistently brought men and women into contact with death and dying, e.g., graves registration, nursing, and body bagging. What is common to these experiences is that the stress with which we are concerned may be the repetition of the experience rather than any particular experience, i.e., the significant stressor may be the cumulative exposure that results in the achievement of a threshold after which stress reactions begin.

The measures of war stress described can all be treated either as discrete events or aggregated into cumulative measures of the veteran's traumatic stress career.[4] The concept of a stress career suggests that frequent exposure to certain types of events produces cumulative stress, and it is more likely to prove a reliable predictor of post-traumatic stress.

An example of this distinction is found in the relationship between killing someone in a war situation and general combat exposure. We found these two variables are highly associated, as would be expected; in the *Legacies of Vietnam* sample the Pearson correlation was 0.57. However, the general measure of combat exposure we developed, which is an additive scale of a range of experiences with a latent measure of the frequency of these events, proves to be a more stable predictor of long-term stress symptomatology and disorder than is the single item variable "killing someone." While some experiences are so graphic and unusual that they have long-term ramifications, such as exposure to acts of abusive violence, others primarily represent a roughly homogeneous class of experiences. Consequently, in terms of experiences like combat, the range of events is more critical to understanding subsequent traumatization than is any particular event. Focusing on specific events, unless they have an exceptional character, proves to be a poorer predictor of long-term stress symptomatology and disorder than measures of cumulative exposure over the war career.[5]

THE SUBJECTIVE RESPONSE TO WAR STRESS

The five elements of war stress described above represent one approach to an understanding of war stress. A second approach involves the subjective responses to external stressors. The significance of retrospectively constructed subjective measures of war stress remains to be considered. There is a broad range of issues involved in the importance of subjective responses to the trauma of war.

Subjective responses to traumatic war stress, we suspect, require a different approach than the cumulative model described above for observable traumatic experiences. The key analytic problem raised by the question of emotional coping is how the process of exposure to stress over time contributes to the development of a dominant subjective coping style to deal with the stressors. By identifying the response to a series of stressors over time, evidence of a dominant coping style for dealing with the death and dying of war may appear. The most reliable subjective predictors of post-traumatic stress symptomatology would expectantly be in the veterans' dominant coping style rather than in their subjective reactions to any particular type of event, such as the death of a friend or the killing of an enemy combatant.

This approach to understanding subjective responses to the death and dying associated with war comes from an analysis which shows that the young men sent to war do not have the repertoire of ego-defenses capable of coping with the warfare society (Laufer, in press). The socialization experience of adolescence and early adulthood in civil society does not provide either a cognitive or emotional guide to the dilemmas posed by war. The ego-mechanisms and emotional responses to war develop in interaction. This process takes time to crystallize. Only by identifying how the early stress is managed and how exposure to subsequent stress influences the emergence of a style of subjective management of stress can reliable emotional predictors of post-traumatic stress be developed.

Evidence shows that generalized subjective responses to war trauma predict post-traumatic symptomatology and disorder (Laufer et al. 1984b). A preliminary analysis examined how coping responses to combat and the death and dying of Americans and Vietnamese are related to post-traumatic stress symptomatology and disorder. However, the measures of coping responses come from open-ended data and reflect general emotional responses to specific stressors rather than general measures of initial and crystallized coping styles discussed above. Nonetheless, some of the findings offer suggestive insights into this issue.

The clearest finding was that numbing the self against the pain of victims, if adopted as a style of coping, is particularly ineffective in dealing with the traumatic experiences of war and tends to result in stress symptomatology and disorder. Some evidence also found that men who acknowledged the pain of victims and their own fears of combat suffered from reexperiencing symptomatology. However, the general range of subjective responses to specific stressful experiences was not significantly related to either stress symptomatology or disorder.

Our interpretation of these findings is twofold. First, stress exposure produces subjective reactions which in turn contribute to heightened vulnerability to subsequent stress. For example, the loss of a friend may lead to acting out, such as killing unarmed civilians or POWs, resulting in more stress exposure (Laufer et al. 1984b). Second, the interaction between stressor exposure and responses to it suggests that the observable measures of stress capture a significant part of the contribution that subjective responses make to post-traumatic stress symptomatology.

STRESS CAREERS

Our conceptualization of war stress can be summarized briefly. Vietnam veterans develop a stress career during their tour of duty. Specifying the elements of that career is a central task of research concerned with the character of post-traumatic stress symptomatology and disorder. The stress career is composed of two elements: (1) distinct and sometimes cumulative classes of observable experiences with external stressors, and (2) subjective responses to individual incidents and experiences which over time lead to the crystallization of a dominant style of coping with the stress of warfare. These two distinct aspects of the stress career lead to two distinct approaches to the measurement of the stressor.

Within each class of observable stressful events we should seek cumulative indices to predict the pattern of stress disorder. The objective in the measurement of subjective stress, on the other hand, is to identify distinct coping styles. Summary measure(s) of subjective coping should reflect the more stable elements of response to stressors. The subjective response to trauma also offers an opportunity to chart the pattern of traumatization in war.

All of these issues cannot be resolved at present. We can, however, demonstrate the significance of both a cumulative approach to stress exposure and the utility of differentiating classes of stressors in identifying the most likely groups to exhibit post-traumatic stress symptomatology and disorder.

The Dimensions of PTSD Symptomatology

A number of models of traumatic neurosis or stress disorder emphasize two dimensions of the response to trauma: (1) a repetition of images, thoughts, and affects from the traumatic event; and (2) defenses against these repetitions (Freud 1953; Lifton and Olson 1976). Horowitz has developed this framework into the most elaborated model of stress disorder. He focuses on the two mental states of (1) "intrusion," which includes intrusive-repetitive thoughts, nightmares, hypervigilance, and pangs of strong emotion; and (2) "denial," which includes inattention, amnesia, constriction of the thought process, and emotional numbing (Horowitz 1976). These two states alternate until the traumatic event is integrated into the individual's world view.

The DSM-III criteria for PTSD include three symptom criteria: (1) Criterion B, "reexperiencing of the trauma," which corresponds to Horowitz's intrusion state; (2) Criterion C, "numbing of responsiveness to the world," which is like Horowitz's avoidance state, being a form of defensiveness although a more severe version of it; and (3) Criterion D, which is a miscellany of symptoms. A close examination of the symptoms in Criterion D reveals that they can be differentiated into symptom clusters that are either subsets of reexperiencing phenomena or defensive maneuvers to avoid it. Thus all three criteria can be organized around the two dimensions of reexperiencing and defensive phenomenon.

In severe forms of traumatic neurosis or stress disorder, clinicians have noted that one or the other of the two dimensions may be dominant (Horowitz 1976). An individual is likely to be overwhelmed with memories, nightmares, and emotions associated with the traumatic event or is likely to be highly defended against such reminders. There is evidence from empirical investigation that one dimension may be dominant at a particular time

Table 1 Measures of Stress Symptomatology and Disorder

Stage 1	Stage 2
The Stress Symptom Inventory	*The Hyperarousal Scale*
1. feelings of dizziness	1. feeling irritable or short-tempered
2. feeling anxious or tense	2. feeling the impulse to lash out
3. headaches	3. occasional feeling of losing control
4. stomach troubles	4. feeling jumpy or easily startled
5. trouble remembering things	5. attacks of sudden fear or panic
6. feeling numb	6. trouble sleeping, staying asleep, or
7. losing interest in usual activities	oversleeping
8. feeling irritable or short tempered	
9. trouble sleeping, staying asleep, or	*The Intrusive Imagery Scale*
oversleeping	1. troubling thoughts about military
10. frightening dreams or nightmares	experiences
11. feeling sad, depressed, or blue	2. frightening dreams or nightmares
12. feeling the impulse to lash out	3. thoughts of how you might die
13. feeling easily tired	
14. occasional feeling of losing control	*The Numbing Scale*
15. feeling jumpy or easily startled	1. losing interest in usual activities
16. attacks of sudden fear or panic	2. feeling that life isn't meaningful
17. thoughts of how you might die	3. feeling that what other people care
18. feeling confused or having trouble	about doesn't make sense
thinking	4. feeling numb
19. trouble trusting others	
20. feeling that life isn't meaningful	*The Cognitive Disruption Scale*
21. troubling thoughts about military	1. feeling confused or having trouble
experiences	thinking
22. feeling that what other people care	2. trouble remembering things
about doesn't make sense	

(Zilberg et al. 1982). Further, evidence also suggests that certain responses to trauma tend to be established early and persist over time in one or the other mode (Laufer et al. 1983a; Hough et al. 1983).

The four columns in Table 1 show the four stages in which we tested the effects of war stress on symptomatology. The initial test concerned whether exposure to war stress increased rates of symptomatology at the time of the interview, well removed from the times at which the men had been exposed to the stressful experiences. Stress symptomatology was measured as an additive scale of the number of symptoms the respondent reported experiencing in the year before the interview. The items in the stress

Table 1 (Continued)

Stage 3	Stage 4
DSM-III	*Dual Stress Disorders*

Stage 3	Stage 4
Diagnostic criteria for Post-traumatic Stress Disorder	

A. Existence of a recognizable stressor that would evoke significant symptoms of distress in almost everyone.	A. The experience of war trauma
	  1. combat experiences
	  2. witnessing of acts of abusive violence
	  3. participation in acts of abusive violence

B. Reexperiencing of the trauma as evidenced by at least one of the following:
  1. recurrent and intrusive recollections of the event
  2. recurrent dreams of the event
  3. sudden acting or feeling as if the traumatic event were recurring, because of an association with an environmental or ideational stimulus
	I. *Disorder Based on Reexperiencing*
	  A. Intrusion
	    1. troubling thoughts about military experiences
	    2. frightening dreams or nightmares
	    3. thoughts of how you might die

C. Numbing of responsiveness to or reduced involvement with the external world, beginning some time after the trauma, as shown by at least one of the following:
  1. markedly diminished interest in one or more significant activities
  2. feeling of detachment or estrangement from others
  3. constricted affect
	B. Hyperarousal
	    1. feeling irritable or short-tempered
	    2. feeling the impulse to lash out
	    3. occasional feeling of losing control
	    4. feeling jumpy or easily startled
	    5. attacks of sudden fear or panic
	    6. trouble sleeping, staying asleep, or oversleeping

D. At least two of the following symptoms that were not present before the trauma:
  1. hyperalertness or exaggerated startle response
  2. sleep disturbance
  3. guilt about surviving when others have not, or about behavior required for survival
  4. memory impairment or trouble concentrating
  5. avoidance of activities that arouse recollection of the traumatic event
  6. intensification of symptoms by exposure to events that symbolize or resemble the traumatic event
	II. *Disorder Based on Denial*
	  A. Numbing
	    1. losing interest in usual activities
	    2. feeling that life isn't meaningful
	    3. feeling that what other people care about doesn't make sense
	    4. feeling numb
	  B. Cognitive Difficulties
	    1. feeling confused or having trouble thinking
	    2. trouble remembering things

symptom inventory list were chosen from the literature on traumatic events and early drafts on the specification of PTSD in DSM-III (Boulanger et al. 1981). Only general combat exposure was found to lead to higher symptom rates among stress-exposed groups (Laufer et al. 1984a).[6]

A more refined test was made by disaggregating the general symptom inventory into four scales based on distinct symptom clusters as shown in stage 2 of Table 1. The pattern of effects found in this test was more complex (Laufer et al. 1983a). Combat exposure contributed to hyperarousal and intrusive imagery symptomatology; witnessing abusive violence contributed to intrusive imagery symptoms; and participation in abusive violence contributed to hyperarousal, numbing, and cognitive disruption symptomatology.

The variation in symptom responses to stress and traumatic experiences shown by this pattern suggested that PTSD may not be the comprehensive phenomenon specified in the DSM-III. To be diagnosed PTSD positive in the current DSM-III formulation, symptoms from each criterion category must be present (at least one each from Criteria B and C, and at least two from Criterion D).

The different linkages between stress exposure and symptom response clusters led to the expectation that PTSD may be a disorder in which one of the two dimensions may dominate the symptom picture. We hypothesized that it may occur as either of two types of response to stress, a reexperiencing- or denial-based form of the disorder. The elements used to construct the measures of reexperiencing and denial-based disorders, and their comparability with the DSM-III specification are shown in stages 3 and 4 of Table 1. The symptom clusters, though not perfectly corresponding to those in the outline of PTSD, were sufficiently comparable to allow a valid test to be made. The limited number of specific symptoms in each cluster, in fact, made the test a conservative one because individuals were less likely to be judged PTSD positive than if the number of symptoms were larger.

The test of the relationship between stress exposure and the two specifications of PTSD showed marked differences in how stress exposure was tied to disorder (Laufer et al. 1983b). Combat exposure was weakly related to the comprehensive specification of disorder, witnessing abusive violence was strongly related to the DSM-III disorder, and participation in abusive violence had no relationship to this disorder. In examining the prevalence rates only a small difference appeared in PTSD positives when comparing low combat veterans (21 percent) and high combat veterans (25 percent).[7] A more sizable difference existed in the rates between those who were not exposed to abusive violence (17 percent) and those who were exposed to acts of abusive violence (29 percent).

In examining the relationship between war stress and the reexperiencing and denial disorders separately there was a significant relationship between combat exposure and the reexperiencing-based disorder, and witnessing abusive violence and the reexperiencing based disorder. Neither of these types of stress exposure was related to the denial-based disorder, however. Participation in abusive violence, on the other hand, was significantly related to denial-based disorder, while having no relationship to the reexperiencing-based disorder.

The prevalence rates showed a clear linear relationship between combat exposure and exhibiting reexperiencing-based disorder. Only 18 percent of low-combat veterans were positive on reexperiencing-based disorder, whereas 31 percent of high-combat veterans were positive on this long-term response. Correspondingly, only 19 percent of men not exposed to abusive violence were positive on reexperiencing-based disorder, while 40 percent of men who witnessed abusive violence were positive. The prevalence rates on denial-based disorder show a similar strong pattern, but only when comparing those who did and did not participate in abusive violence. Only 19 percent of veterans who did not participate in abusive violence were positive on denial-based disorder; 43 percent of veterans who did participate were positive.

The DSM-III diagnosis of PTSD appears to be limited in two ways. First, the DSM-III model of PTSD clearly biases diagnosis of disorder toward those who report reexperiencing symptoms. Second, only those who combine reexperiencing with denial symptoms are likely to fall into the diagnostic category under the current disorder. Thus, even the reexperiencing prevalence estimate is low within the context of the current diagnostic guidelines.

CONCLUSION

Two fundamental points in our discussion deserve special emphasis. First, we believe that the conceptualization of war stress at present is not sufficiently developed to empirically determine all of the long-term effects of war trauma on the lives of veterans. Unless the nature of war stressors is more systematically addressed along the lines we have suggested, diagnosis and research will continue to be hampered in identifying the presence of PTSD in the Vietnam veteran population. This problem will best be resolved by taking into account three issues in developing a war stress model: (1) the cumulative character of war stress; (2) the differentiation of classes of stressors; and (3) the relationship between objective stressors and the development of subjective coping styles. Second, our analysis also points to the importance of reconceptualizing the symptomatological configurations associated with PTSD. The finding that there is a consistent relationship between distinct aspects of disorder and certain war stressors suggests that a more flexible approach to disorder, one which acknowledges that either reexperiencing- or denial-based PTSD may dominate the symptom picture, should be followed. These issues require further research and discussion so that PTSD can be more carefully specified and validly and reliably identified.

References

American Psychiatric Association: Diagnostic and Statistical Manual of Mental Disorders, 3rd ed. Washington, DC, American Psychiatric Association, 1980

Boulanger G, Kadushin C, Martin J: Legacies of Vietnam, vol IV. Long Term Stress Reactions. Washington, DC, US Government Printing Office, 1981

Brett B: Imagery and post-traumatic stress disorder. West Haven, Conn, VAMC Merit Review Study, 1983

Card JJ: Lives After Vietnam: The Personal Impact of Military Service. Lexington, Mass, Lexington Books, 1983

Figley C (ed.): Stress Disorders Among Vietnam Veterans. New York, Brunner/Mazel, 1978

Foy DW, Research Team: Vietnam Veterans Readjustment Research Project, Working Papers. Brentwood, Calif, Veterans Administration, 1981

Freud S: Beyond the pleasure principle (1921), in Complete Psychological Works, standard ed, vol 18. Translated and edited by Strachey J. London, Hogarth Press, 1953

Grinker RR, Spiegel JP: Men Under Stress. Philadelphia, Blakiston, 1945

Harris L: Myths and Realities: A Study of Attitudes Toward Vietnam Era Veterans. Washington, DC, US Government Printing Office, 1980

Horowitz MJ: Stress Response Syndromes. New York, Jason Aronson, 1976

Hough R, Gongla PA, Scurfield RM et al: Natural history of post-traumatic stress disorder. Paper presented at American Psychological Association, Anaheim, Calif, 1983

Kardiner A, Spiegel H: War Stress and Neurotic Illness. New York, Hoeber, 1947

Krystal H, Niederland WG: Psychic Traumatization. Boston, Little Brown, 1971

Laufer RS: War trauma and human developments: Vietnam, in Psychiatric Affects of the Vietnam War. Edited by Sonnenberg S, Blank A, Talbot J (in press)

Laufer RS, Gallops MS: The effects of war trauma on life course development. Paper presented at American Sociological Association, Detroit, 1983

Laufer RS, Brett E, Gallops MS: Dimensions of post-traumatic stress among Vietnam veterans. Paper presented at American Psychiatric Association, New York, 1983a

Laufer RS, Brett E, Gallops MS: Patterns of post-traumatic stress disorder among Vietnam veterans exposed to combat and abusive violence. Paper presented at American Psychological Association, New York, 1983b

Laufer RS, Gallops MS, Frey-Wouters E: War stress and post-war trauma. J Health Soc Behav (in press), 1984a

Laufer RS, Frey-Wouters E, Gallops, MS: Traumatic stressors in the Vietnam war and post-traumatic stress disorder, in Trauma and its Wake. Edited by Figley C (in press), 1984b

Laufer RS, Yager T, Frey-Wouters E, et al: Legacies of Vietnam, vol III. Post-War Trauma: Social and Psychological Problems of Vietnam Veterans and Their Peers. Washington, DC, US Government Printing Office, 1981

Lifton RJ, Olson E: The human meaning of total disaster: the Buffalo Creek experience. Psychiatry 39:1–18, 1976

Moskos C: The American Enlisted Man. New York, Russell Sage, 1970

Polk K: The Marion County youth study. Eugene, Ore, National Institute of Mental Health, 1980

Rothbart G: Legacies of Vietnam, vol II. General Methodology:79–97. Washington, DC, US Government Printing Office, 1981

Stouffer SA, Lumsdaine AA, Lumsdaine MH, et al: The American Soldier, vol II. Combat and Its Aftermath. Princeton, Princeton University Press, 1949

Wheaton B: Stress, personal coping resources, and psychiatric symptoms: an investigation of interactive models. J Health Soc Behav 24:208–229, 1983

Wilson J, Krauss GE: Vietnam Era Stress Inventory. Cleveland, Cleveland State University, 1980

Wilson J, Krauss GE: Predicting post-traumatic stress syndromes among Vietnam veterans. Paper presented at 25th Neuropsychiatric Institute, VA Medical Center, Coatesville, Pa, 1982

Yager T, Laufer RS, Gallops MS: Some problems associated with war experience in men of the Vietnam generation. Arch Gen Psychiatry (in press)

Zilberg NJ, Weiss DS, Horowitz MJ: Impact of event scale: a cross-validational study and some empirical evidence supporting a conceptual model of stress response syndromes. J Consult Clin Psychol 50:407–414, 1982

Notes

[1] Our data are derived from the *Legacies of Vietnam* study commissioned by the Veteran's Administration to investigate the psychological, behavioral and social impact of military service during the Vietnam conflict. A probability sample of 1,342 men was collected from ten sites matched on economic and demographic characteristics, from four sections of the country, the northeast, south, midwest and west. Besides geography, the sample was also stratified on the basis of veteran status, race, and age. The sample contained 350 Vietnam veterans, 363 veterans who served in the same period but not in Vietnam, and 629 nonveterans (Rothbart 1981). The data on war stress and post-traumatic stress disorder presented in this paper are based on the analysis of the 350 Vietnam veterans.

[2] The combat scale we developed is composed of ten items: 1. Served in an artillery unit which fired on the enemy; 2. Flew in an aircraft over Vietnam; 3. Stationed at a forward observation post; 4. Received incoming fire; 5. Encountered mines or booby traps; 6. Received sniper or sapper fire; 7. In a patrol which was ambushed; 8. Engaged VC or NVA in a firefight; 9. Saw Americans or Vietnamese killed; and 10. Was

wounded. The scale was coded in an additive fashion. Items 1 through 6 were given a value of 1 if true, items 7 through 10 were given a value of 2 if true. The value of each experience was added cumulatively. The maximum range on the scale was from (0)—"Had none of these experiences," to (14)—"Had all of these experiences." The effective range of the scale in our sample was (0) to (13). The mean of the scale was 5.9; the median 5.7; and the standard deviation 4.1 (the characteristics of the weighted data). Nine percent of the sample saw no combat, 33 percent saw low combat (values 1 through 4), 31 percent saw moderate combat (values 5 through 9), and 27 percent saw heavy combat (values 10 through 13).

[3] In measuring exposure to abusive violence we used a set of open-ended questions in which the veteran was asked whether he experienced the dirty side of war and to describe the events in this category. We required that veterans had at least witnessed the event or had seen its consequences soon after its commission and had clearly known who had carried it out. To make the measure an indicator of objective experiences we eliminated any events of which they had heard second hand. In our sample, roughly a third (31 percent) reported they were directly exposed to at least one episode. These episodes varied in character, but the most often cited were the torture of prisoners, including pushing them from helicopters; the physical mistreatment of civilians; the use of napalm, white phosphorus, or cluster bombs on villages; death or maiming by booby trap; and the mutilation of bodies. Most of the men who reported episodes described cases in which U.S. regulars were involved (78 percent of those exposed). Less than a third mentioned ones in which the Viet Cong or North Vietnamese regulars were involved (31 percent of those exposed). Another 13 percent reported cases in which Army of the Republic of Vietnam (ARVN) or Korean (ROK) forces were involved. (These three figures do not sum to 100 percent since over a third of those exposed mentioned more than one episode.) In previous work we tested a model which differentiated the effects of exposure to abusive violence by the perpetrator of the act. Our findings suggest that the traumatic quality of the experience is the imagery associated with it; the issue of who initiated the action was not significant if the veteran had only witnessed the event and did not participate in it personally. Consequently, the emphasis in constructing measures of abusive violence should be on the

distinction between those who witnessed episodes and those who actively participated in them.

[4] Another aspect of military service which has received attention as contributing to subsequent stress reactions is serving multiple tours. Foy's data (1980) suggest that the length of time a veteran spent in Vietnam has a very powerful effect on long-term adjustment. Multiple tours of duty are relatively rare, but in those cases where individuals have more than one tour, especially where there are more than two tours, the evidence suggests significant increases in symptomatology and behavioral problems. It is extremely likely that a measure of multiple tours simply reflects a greater range and frequency of exposure to other stress experiences. If such is the case then serving multiple tours would not be stressful in and of itself, but would appear so if other measures of stress exposure were not controlled.

[5] Measures of the witnessing of and participation in abusive violence, though dichotomous in form, are not based on the assumption that we are measuring a single experience's effect on subsequent stress symptomatology. Frequently, men who reported witnessing abusive violence commonly saw more than a single event; and even among the participants, our transcript material indicates that it is not uncommon for these men to have participated in more than one such action. The use of a dichotomous measure is a function of restrictions in the data of the *Legacies* study. In ongoing research the impact of multiple exposures or participation in abusive violence is being examined (Brett 1983).

[6] See note 4.

[7] Low combat exposure is defined as a score of 0 to 4 on the combat scale (33 percent of the Vietnam veteran sample). High combat exposure is defined as a score of 10 to 13 on the combat scale (27 percent of the Vietnam veteran sample).

5

The Dream Experience in Dream-Disturbed Vietnam Veterans

Milton Kramer, M.D.
Lawrence S. Schoen, Ph.D.
Lois Kinney, Ph.D.

5

The Dream Experience
in Dream-Disturbed
Vietnam Veterans

Interest in post-traumatic stress disorder (PTSD), traumatic neurosis, is currently high and comes from three sources. The first source of our increased interest is the recognition that PTSD occurred frequently among veterans of the Vietnam War (Figley 1978). The second source of our interest stems from our appreciation that survivors of civilian disasters, such as the collapse of the dam at Buffalo Creek, have had considerable and continuing psychological distress following their experience (Gieser et al. 1981). And, third, at the individual level, there is a continuing concern about victims of industrial accidents (Group for the Advancement of Psychiatry 1977) and rape (Burgess and Holstrom 1974) who develop both acute and delayed PTSD.

With the recognition of the increased frequency of patients suffering from PTSD, the concept of PTSD has been defined more carefully and specifically in the third edition of the *Diagnostic and Statistical Manual of Mental Disorders* (DSM-III) (American Psychiatric Association 1980). The diagnostic criteria for PTSD have four components. The first is the existence of a recognizable stressor. The second is the reexperiencing of the trauma, by either (a) recurring intrusive recollections of the event, (b) recurring dreams of the event, or (c) sudden acting or feeling as if the event were occurring. The third component of PTSD is a numbing of responsiveness to or a reduced involvement with the external world beginning after the trauma, and possibly including (a) diminished interest in significant activities, (b) feelings of detachment or estrangement, and (c) constricted affect. Last, at least two of the following symptoms must be present subsequent to the trauma: (a) hyperalertness (startle), (b) sleep disturbance, (c) survivor's guilt, (d) problems with memory and concentration, (e) avoiding situations that arouse the traumatic memory, and (f) having symbols of the trauma stir up the symptoms.

Disturbed dreaming may be the hallmark of delayed PTSD (Kramer 1979). Boulanger's data points out that disturbed dreaming is highly correlated with and more frequent than waking reexperiencing of the traumatic event in PTSD sufferers (Boulanger G: A measurement of traumatic stress reactions developed in a probability sample of Vietnam veterans, era veterans, and nonveterans. Unpublished manuscript, 1980). Since reexperiencing the traumatic event during wakefulness or sleep is one of the four criteria necessary to make a diagnosis of PTSD, disturbing dreams relating to the traumatic event may truly be at the center of the disorder.

Because of the frequent identification of patients suffering from PTSD in Veterans Administration (VA) hospitals, there is an increasing need to examine systematically various aspects of the disorder. The identification of biological and psychological correlates of the disorder would facilitate identification of PTSD sufferers for treatment and research purposes (Sierles et al. 1983) as well as sort out potential malingerers from bona fide cases (Sparr and Pankratz 1983). A study of the dreams of PTSD sufferers may provide insights into the nature of the disorder.

Freud discussed the central role of dreams in traumatic neuroses and felt that these dreams were a challenge to his wish fulfillment theory of dreaming (Freud 1920). Dreams were seen as the protector of sleep by Freud; yet in traumatic neuroses, they appeared to be the disturber of sleep. He finally came to the conclusion that the disturbing dream was an exception to his theory and that, in fact, the dream in traumatic neuroses was an effort at mastering the stress of the traumatic experience.

Counselling efforts which focus on reliving and reexperiencing the Vietnam War experience reflect an acceptance of Freud's position (Keane and Fairbank 1983). Certainly, many veterans of the Vietnam War, once their confidence is won, do focus on the reexperiencing of war-related events, both awake and asleep.

Modern dream research has expanded Freud's view of traumatic dreaming and has noted that two types of terrifying arousals are present out of sleep. These arousals are probably stage-dependent events. Broughton (1968) has described night terrors, arousals out of deep sleep early in the night, which fit the description of incubus or pavor nocturnus. In these experiences the individual is terrified and exhibits autonomic activation. Accompanying these arousals, within ten seconds, are heart rate increases from 60 to 100 beats per minute (bpm) and respiratory rate increases from 20 to 40 breaths per minute. In a severe episode the sufferer often awakens sweating, his pupils are dilated, and his accompanying mental content for the event is essentially nil. This sequence of events is in contrast to frightening arousals out of rapid eye movement (REM) sleep—dream anxiety attacks—which were described by Fischer (1974). In these instances there may or may not be autonomic arousal, and there is considerably more elaborated dream content.

It was apparent, given our current understanding of the two different physiological and behavioral categories of disturbing dreams, that dream-disturbed individuals with PTSD would have to be studied based on these two distinguishing characteristics; namely, those who had a preponderance of non-REM-disturbed dreaming (night terrors) and those who had a preponderance of REM-disturbed dreaming (dream anxiety attacks). It is perfectly possible that individuals who manifest each of these types of disturbing dreams belong to a single population. Initially, however, they should be treated as two separate groups.

Other aspects of the disturbed dream sufferer, whether manifesting night terrors/nightmare or dream anxiety attacks, have to be taken into account. Some have the condition lifelong, and some develop it in adult life. Hartman has suggested that those with lifelong disturbing dreams are potentially quite ill psychologically

(Hartman et al. 1981) and have poorly differentiated self-boundaries (Hartman et al. 1983).

The time course of the disturbed dreaming in relationship to the trauma is another factor to be taken into account in studying disturbed dreaming. Post-traumatic stress disorder has been described in an acute form, coming on right after the trauma; and in a delayed form, coming on some six months or more after the trauma (Boulanger, unpublished manuscript, 1980). The delayed form may have been preceded by an acute form of the disorder that may or may not have resolved. In studying disturbed dreaming, these time dimensions must be specified because the personality and sleep and dream patterns may be different in the two conditions.

We examined disturbed dreamers who are Vietnam combat veterans and compared their recall of their combat experience, their personality structure, their clinical diagnoses, and their sleep and dreams with a group of Vietnam combat veterans who did not complain about disturbed dreaming. This approach facilitated our understanding of the possible role of disturbed dreaming in PTSD.

METHOD

The subjects were solicited by newspaper advertisement and by requests from colleagues for referral. We were seeking two comparable groups of Vietnam combat veterans. One group had to have a disturbed dream frequency of once per week; the other group, the control group, had to have no disturbed dreaming.

To control for illness, the control group had to have at least one of Boulanger's six threshold symptoms: (1) trouble remembering, (2) loss of interest, (3) feelings of loss of control, (4) panic attacks, and (5) periods of confusion. The control group could not have disturbed dreaming, the sixth symptom, as a complaint. These are the symptoms that are most frequently reported by Vietnam veterans who have PTSD.

The subjects answering the advertisement were interviewed to obtain a sleep/dream history. They also went through a diagnostic procedure that included the administration of the Schedule for

Table 1 Dream Recall and Content During Nights 1–4

	DD (n = 7)			Control (n = 8)		
	Total	REM	non-REM	Total	REM	non-REM
Awakenings	3.3	0.7	2.6	2.2	0.4	1.8
Awakenings with Content	1.8	0.5	1.3	1.0	0.2	0.8
Percentage Dream Recall	55%	77%	50%	45%	50%	44%
Dreams with Military References	0.8	0.25	0.57	0.03	0.0	0.03
Percentage of Dreams with Military References	44%	50%	44%	3%	0	4%

Affective Diseases and Schizophrenia (SADS), the Minnesota Multiphasic Personality Inventory (MMPI), and an evaluation for PTSD using the Traumatic Stress Reaction Scale and the criteria from DSM-III needed to make a diagnosis of PTSD. Personality assessments were done at the trait and state level. Trait assessment included four measures of trait anxiety (The Cornell Medical Index [CMI], Taylor Manifest Anxiety Scale, Spielberger Trait Anxiety Scale, and the Pt Scale of the MMPI), three measures of depression (the D Scale of the MMPI, the Depression Scale of the CMI, and the Beck Depression Inventory), and one measure of locus of control (Rotter I-E Scale). The state assessments included the Spielberger Anxiety Scale and the Clyde Mood Scale, both of which were administered before and after each night the subject slept in the laboratory. In addition, combat experience was assessed using the Combat Inventory Scales of the Vietnam Era Stress Inventory.

The subject then slept for six consecutive nights in the laboratory. On the first four nights, each time the subject awakened for more than one minute, there was an inquiry about what was going through his mind (dream). On night five, the subject was, in addition, awakened twice from each sleep stage and dream data were collected. Night six was a sleep-through night, and no dream data were obtained.

Subjects were asked to rate on a one- to five-point scale the fear and anxiety associated with each dream experience at the time the dream was obtained. If the dream was rated three or four on either scale, it was considered a disturbing dream. If they had more disturbing dreams out of non-REM than REM, they were placed in the dream-disturbed group. The control group had no disturbed dreaming. Each night and morning in the laboratory additional information about the subject's experience was gathered. This included measures of personal feelings and stress.

RESULTS

Table 1 shows the results reported in this section.

Awakenings

Across the four nights of spontaneous awakenings, the mean number of dream report awakenings for each subject in the dream-disturbed group (DD) was 13 and for the control group (C) it was 9. Therefore, there were 3.3 awakenings in the dream-disturbed group and 2.2 awakenings in the control group per night.

In the dream-disturbed group, 79 percent of the awakenings came from non-REM sleep, while 21 percent came out of REM sleep. In the control group, the awakenings were distributed 82 percent from non-REM and 18 percent from REM. The two groups had approximately the same distribution of REM and non-REM sleep. REM sleep in both groups comprised 16 percent of the night while the percentage of time spent in non-REM sleep was 69 percent and 71 percent for the dream-disturbed and control groups, respectively. Therefore, awakenings were distributed proportionately to the distribution of REM and non-REM sleep in the night.

Dream Reports

In the dream-disturbed group 1.8 awakenings with dreams occurred per subject per night; in the control group 1.0 awakenings with dreams occurred per subject per night. The dream recall rate was 55 percent for the dream disturbed and 45 percent for the control group. When the stage of sleep was examined as it was related to dream recall from an awakening, the DD group had a 77 percent recall of dream content from awakenings out of REM and 50 percent out of non-REM. The control group had 50 percent recall from REM awakenings and 44 percent from non-REM.

Military Dream Content

How many of the dream reports made direct reference to any military experience? There was an average of 0.8 dreams with military reference per subject per night in the dream-disturbed group and 0.03 in the control group. Dreams with military references on the average made up 47 percent of the dream reports of the DD group and only 4 percent of the dream reports of the control group.

The stage of sleep out of which the dream came played no role in whether the dream had a military reference. In the DD group 50 percent of the REM dreams had a military reference and, 44 percent of the non-REM dreams had a military reference. In the control group, there were essentially no military references in any recalled dreams.

DISCUSSION

During the night, 50 percent more spontaneous awakenings were identified in the dream-disturbed group than in the control group. However, when the records were scored later, it turned out that the two groups had essentially the same number of spontaneous awakenings. The dream-disturbed group had nine awakenings per night and the control group had eight awakenings. Therefore, the initial differences in spontaneous awakenings found between the two groups likely were due to the experimenter's inability to identify one minute of stage wake during the night. Clearly, it was easier to identify awakenings in the dream-disturbed than in the control group. This may be due to the awakenings being 15 percent longer in the dream-disturbed group. This increased ease of identification accounts for the dream-disturbed group having 3.3 awakenings per night while the control group had 2.2

The distribution of awakenings between REM and non-REM sleep reflect the amount of non-REM and REM sleep the two groups actually obtained. The dream-disturbed group and the control group both had 19 percent of their sleep time in REM and 81 percent of their sleep time in non-REM. This mirrors almost identically the distribution of awakenings from REM and non-REM in the two groups. Therefore, the possibility of an awakening being identified by the experimenters is not different between the two stages of sleep. However, awakenings and arousals do occur more often in the dream-disturbed subjects during non-REM sleep in the first half of the night (Kinney 1983). This shift in distribution of awakenings and arousals did not influence identification of awakenings from which dream recall was obtained.

The probability of a dream recalled from an awakening was not different between the two groups. Because the awakenings were from both REM and non-REM sleep, the overall recall percentages of 55 percent and 45 percent for the two groups are about what one might expect (Foulkes 1966). However, when recall rates are looked at as a function of the stage of sleep out of which they occurred, one finds a difference between the groups. In the dream-disturbed group, the recall of a dream occurs from 77 percent of awakenings out of REM sleep; while in the control group, it only occurs 50 percent of the time. Further, non-REM recall is about the same in the two groups (50 percent and 44 percent) and not different from what has been reported elsewhere from non-REM dreaming (Foulkes 1966). Yet, the dream-disturbed group was selected for the greater recall and experience of disturbing dreams out of non-REM sleep in the laboratory.

The difference in the recall between the two groups of dream events out of REM sleep might be due to a difference in personality orientation of the two groups. It is possible that the dream-disturbed group is indeed having more disturbing dreams and is indeed more focused on internal processes which are disturbing. The dream recall rate is not excessive, but it is what one would expect from REM-period awakenings (Snyder 1969).

The control group, which has a lower than normal recall rate from REM sleep, is one that clearly is not attending to inner processes. They are, based on personality indices, a relatively less troubled group. They are not focused on their dream experience and may actually not be attending to inner processes. This may be a "healthier adaptation" or be the avoidance of inner processes as a way of making an adaptation. Indeed, there were indications that subjects in the control group had more symptoms of PTSD immediately following their military experience than they are now experiencing.

When one looks at the presence of dreams with military references, one sees a clear difference between the two groups. Military references occur in 44 percent of the recalled dreams of the dream-disturbed group but in only 4 percent of the dreams recalled by the control group. When looked at from a sleep stage point of view, the dreams with military references occur with equal frequency out of both REM and non-REM sleep.

Although selected for dream disturbances predominantly out of non-REM sleep, the dream-disturbed group has an equal percentage of military-related content in both REM and non-REM dreams. This suggests that their mental content during sleep is not stage dependent, and that the pervasive nature of the mental content may play a fundamental role in sustaining the traumatic state. Thus, disturbing mental content is potentially available as a sleep disrupter at all times of the night.

It is interesting to speculate about the occurrence of military dreams in the present situation. The combat veterans without disturbing dreams do not have military-related dreams; the combat veterans with dream disturbances clearly do. Further, their military dreams are as likely to occur out of non-REM sleep as they are out of REM sleep. This suggests that the preoccupation with the military is not bound to one part of the night and is a continuing focus for the dream-disturbed combat veteran.

The presence of military dreams is one, if not the only, feature which distinguishes combat veterans from non-disturbed dreamer veterans in an all or none matter. This lends further credence to our view that the dream disturbance may be central to the pathological process in PTSD. That is, the disturbing dream may continually reinforce the traumatic neurosis. One should keep in mind, however, that only 50 percent of the dreams in the dream-disturbed group actually have a military reference. Therefore, there are other areas of importance in the lives of these subjects than simply the military experience. This is a fact that might well have to be taken into account in any treatment approach to this group.

If the dream reflects the current emotional focus of the dreamer (Kramer 1982), then clearly the dream-disturbed subjects and the control group have different foci. The dream-disturbed group is clearly more focused around military issues, and for them, this means Vietnam. However, there is a large segment of dream life that does not involve military issues. The treatment approaches that focus exclusively on the Vietnam experience will not attend to the other areas of importance in the patient's life. It is not that there is no concern about the war, it is just that it is not the only concern that the patient has. The impression that one might draw is that there are concerns about both areas and that, perhaps, they are interrelated. It is worthwhile to try to illustrate the point.

CASE EXAMPLE

A Vietnam veteran had volunteered to sleep in the Dream/Sleep Laboratory at the VA Hospital. He felt stalemated in his therapeutic work on his problems. Two years previously his wife had left him, and following that, he became more and more troubled and preoccupied with his Vietnam experience. Approximately four months before sleeping in the laboratory, he had quit his job and returned his gun to his boss for fear of getting into difficulty. A brief synopsis of his five dreams collected during one night in the laboratory follows.

Dream 1: He was trying to cross a river and a big guy was trying to help him. It seemed that they were in the Mekong Delta. Every time they tried to get to the other side, they were back at the beginning.

Dream 2: He was a young boy at home and was fighting with

one of the neighborhood kids. His brother was around. The kid they were fighting was one who later died in Vietnam.

Dream 3: He went with others to a construction site. He was a sapper, like in Vietnam. He blew the site up. The consequence of blowing up the construction site was that his brother's house was flooded.

Dream 4: He remembers being a young child in his parent's home. There was some argument and he left. He wrote them postcards without a forwarding address. Every time they would try to contact him, he had moved somewhere else.

Dream 5: He was driving very fast, and his wife was worried that he would have an accident.

The patient was surprised by the focus on his family and his wife. Prior to his laboratory experience he didn't think that his family was an issue. Following the experience in the laboratory, he went back and sought out his wife to see if there could be a reconciliation. His work with his therapist was rejuvenated as he worked on both past and current problems.

This brief illustration suggests an interaction between the past and the present and between the military and nonmilitary experiences of the patient's life. It is striking that 60 percent of the dreams are military and 40 percent are nonmilitary, similar to that found in our PTSD veterans.

Again, assuming that the dream reflects the current concern of the individual, a great deal of the personal concern of the dream-disturbed patient is on matters not obviously related to the traumatic experience. It will be interesting to see if the group selected for greater REM disturbed dreaming than non-REM disturbed dreaming reflects a similar pattern. One might predict that this would indeed be the case because the dream-disturbed group tended to have an equal percentage of military content in the REM and non-REM dreams.

We suggest that attention to the current and past situation is necessary in the treatment of PTSD victims as their dreams are focused on the traumatic event and other problematic areas in their lives.

Two previous attempts to study PTSD in war victims in the sleep laboratory (Lavie et al. 1979; Schlosberg and Benjamin 1978) were done in Israel. Neither of them was able to study subjects with frequent and documented dream disturbances, and neither obtained systematic dream reports. Therefore, this is the first systematic study of dream reports obtained in the laboratory of subjects with dream disturbances secondary to a war experience and compared to appropriate controls.

Note should be made that the groups in this study were not selected for PTSD. Rather, they were combat veterans of the Vietnam War who were selected for either a high or low frequency of disturbing dreams. High frequency of disturbing dreams does indeed correlate highly with the diagnosis of PTSD in the present study. We found that eight out of eight of our disturbed dreamers had PTSD while only one out of eight of the control group had PTSD. Disturbed dreaming may well turn out to be at the core of the PTSD.

CONCLUSIONS

The dreams of the Vietnam veteran with disturbed dreaming are indeed different than his combat peer without disturbed dreaming. Both awakened frequently and overall recalled their dreams at about the same rate. However, the control group tended to have a lower rate of dream recall from REM awakenings. This suggests that the control group may be coping by avoiding potentially disturbing experiences represented in dreams.

The dreams of patients with disturbed dreaming tend to have a military theme in about half of their dreams, while practically none of the dreams of the control group are military related. Military dreams occur in equal proportion out of both REM and non-REM sleep, despite the dream-disturbed group being selected for a preponderance of bad dreams out of non-REM.

The dream experience, its intensity (recallability), content, and distribution may well lie at the heart of PTSD. The disturbing dream may continually reinforce the traumatic neuroses.

References

Broughton R: Sleep disorders: disorders of arousal? Science 159:1070–1078, 1968

Burgess A, Holmstrom L: Rape: victims of crisis. Bowie, Md, Robert J Brady, 1974, pp 44–47

Figley CR (ed.): Stress Disorders among Vietnam Veterans: Theory, Research and Treatment. New York, Brunner/Mazel, 1978

Fischer C, Kahn E, Edwards A, et al: A psychophysiological study of nightmares and night terrors. Psychoanal Contemp Sci 3:317–398, 1974

Foulkes D: The Psychology of Sleep. New York, Charles Scribner's Sons, 1966

Freud S: Beyond the Pleasure Principle (1920), in Complete Psychological Works, standard ed, vol 18. Translated and edited by Strachey J. London, Hogarth Press, 1955

Gieser GC, Green BL, Winget CN: Prolonged Psychological Effects of a Disaster: Buffalo Creek. New York, Academic Press, 1981

Group for the Advancement of Psychiatry, Committee on Psychiatry in Industry: What Price Compensation? GAP Report No. 99. Group for the Advancement of Psychiatry, 1977

Hartman E, Russ D, van der Kolk B, et al: A preliminary study of the personality of the nightmare sufferer: relationship to schizophrenia and creativity. Am J Psychiatry 138:794–797, 1981

Hartman E, Sivan I, Cooper S, et al: The personality of lifelong nightmare sufferers: projective test results. Paper presented at the Fourth International Congress of Sleep Research, Bologna, Italy, 1983

Keane TM, Fairbank JA: Survey analysis of combat-related disorders in Vietnam veterans. Am J Psychiatry 140:348–350, 1983

Kinney L: A laboratory investigation of changes in sleep physiology in the dream-disturbed. Unpublished Doctoral Dissertation, 1983

Kramer M: Dream disturbances. Psychiatric Annals 9:50–68, 1979

Kramer M: The psychology of the dream: art or science? Psych J Univ Ottawa 7:87–100, 1982

Lavie P, Hefez A, Halperin G, et al: Long-term effects of traumatic war-related events on sleep. Am J Psychiatry 136:175–178, 1979

Schlosberg A, Benjamin M: Sleep patterns in three acute combat fatigue cases. J Clin Psychiatry 39:546–549, 1978

Sierles FS, Chen JJ, McFarland, et al: Posttraumatic stress disorder and concurrent psychiatric illness: a preliminary report. Am J Psychiatry 140:1177–1179, 1983

Snyder F: The physiology of dreaming, in Dream Psychology and The New Biology of Dreaming. Edited by Kramer M. Springfield, Ill, Charles C Thomas, pp 7–37, 1969

Sparr L, Pankratz LD: Factitious posttraumatic stress disorder. Am J Psychiatry 140:1016–1019, 1983

6

Propranolol and Clonidine in Treatment of the Chronic Post-Traumatic Stress Disorders of War

Lawrence C. Kolb, M.D.
B. Cullen Burris, M.D.
Susan Griffiths, R.N.

6

Propranolol and Clonidine in Treatment of the Chronic Post-Traumatic Stress Disorders of War

POST-TRAUMATIC STRESS DISORDER AS A CONDITIONED EMOTIONAL RESPONSE

The existence of a subgroup of Vietnam combat veterans suffering from chronic post-traumatic stress disorder (PTSD) who have a conditioned emotional response assumed to be the driving force in (1) maintaining certain constant symptoms of the condition and (2) preventing resolution of the secondarily evolved avoidance behavior and neurotic outlays has been suggested in data collected by Kolb (1982). These data were derived from clinical research, still ongoing, conducted in collaboration with Professor E. Blanchard and his associates T.P. Pallmeyer and R.J. Gerardi, of the Stress Laboratory of the State University of New York at Albany. In this project, psychophysiological responses of a group of combat veterans with clinical symptoms of chronic PTSD were compared with a same aged group of nonveterans without such symptoms. When exposed to a short burst of meaningful combat sounds, played at varying intensities, all but one veteran displayed significant increases in heart rate, systolic blood pressure, and forehead muscle activity, whereas the control group did not. Exposure to other sounds did not produce such responses. The one veteran exception, who at that time was taking the psychopharmaceutic agent, haldol, also stated the sound track was unrealistic to him. On a mental arithmetic stress test the physiological responses of both groups were similar. This work is being pursued. Physiological assessments to similar stimuli are now under examination in other control groups including noncombatant Vietnam-era veterans, noncombatant Vietnam-era veterans who served in Vietnam, and civilians diagnosed as suffering chronic anxiety disorders. To date the new data support the earlier findings of the differential responsiveness to combat sounds of those with diagnosed PTSD. The findings corroborate the earlier report by Dodds and Wilson (1960) that a conditioned emotional response exists in combat veterans of World War II (WWII) who suffered chronic post-traumatic stress disorders.

Preceding the above laboratory observations, a series of narcosynthetic therapeutic trials noted that 14 of 18 Vietnam veterans with PTSD immediately time regressed and reenacted a traumatic scene on exposure to a similar tape of combat sounds. Thus, not all combat veterans who present with the clinical symptomatology of PTSD exhibit evidence of emotional conditioning. From these findings we have postulated an enduring potential for pathophysiological arousal of self-preservative emotions in the chronic and delayed forms of PTSD. This arousal occurs when confronted with either an external stimuli signaling threat, or, when through actual or fantasized social transactions that induce associated threat affects, the affects contained in the conditioned emotional response (fear, rage, or hopeless despair) and/or their secondary elaborations in guilty or shameful anxiety are aroused.

It is interesting that the concept of "conditioning" as a primary driving force in the maintenance of chronic post-traumatic states of war was proposed by Kardiner (1947) as a result of his extended clinical studies of WWI veterans, and that this was reported prior to WWII. Kardiner was impressed by the persistence of startle responses and irritability. The other four major features of post-traumatic states induced by combat experience were (2) fixation on the trauma, (3) atypical dream life, (4) proclivity to explosive reactions, and (5) constriction of the general level of personality functioning. To him, the etiologic issue differed from the ordinary social neurosis in that the problem related to impairment of personality functions concerned with adaptation of the sufferers to the real external world; rather than the ordinary neurosis where psychological conflicts are concerned more with adaptation to and between inner world representations of humanity and society. Kardiner coined the term "physioneurosis" to identify this condition, in contrast to an older term, "actual neurosis," used by Freud (1919).

In the paper describing our experiences we expressed two facets in the severely impaired: (1) a persisting potential for abnormal physiological arousal to any perceived bodily threat and the related emotion state (a physioneurosis); and (2) secondary attempts at adaptation both to the disturbed perception of self as well as to existing and preexisting social representations. In our therapeutic work using individual and group psychotherapy—including hypnosis narcosynthesis, pharmacotherapy, and also desensitization—we have yet to observe persisting relief from the so-called constant symptoms of (to use modern terminology) irritability, explosiveness, repetitive dreams, and intrusive thoughts of the traumatic events. Attempts at desensitization to meaningful threatening sounds failed miserably, as the seven men so exposed were never able to reduce the sound effects to levels where they did not experience arousal of some distressing physiological symptoms. The lack of reports from those who similarly attempted sound deconditioning for startle in WWII veterans with PTSD suggests that those attempts also ended in failure. Furthermore, studies of the literature on treatment of those with the survivors' syndrome of the concentration camps suggest very limited success in alleviation of the persistent symptoms; although none of the writers clearly delineates targeted symptoms, nor focuses upon change in such symptoms, as an indication of progress from therapeutic intervention.

PTSD AND THE NORADRENERGIC SYSTEM

Our clinical experiences, then, and review of that of others treating the chronic and delayed forms of PTSD have led us to the hypothesis that evidence of a persisting conditioned emotional response does exist in the groups of PTSD sufferers. Treatment progress will require blocking or measurable attenuation of the emotional response. Furthermore, the emotional arousal observed in the identified patients presumably is related to abnormalities in the central adrenergic system—either as a result of excessive secretion or enduring hypersensitivity at receptors consequent to a resetting of the discharge potential. The use of psychopharmacological agents will most successfully block this system.

In light of the assumption that the increase in pulse rate, systolic blood pressure, and muscle tension were due to sympathetic neuronal discharge, we decided to attempt a therapeutic trial of several adrenergic blocking agents, particularly propranolol. Beta blockers now have been prescribed successfully in the treatment of performance anxiety in musicians (Neftel et al. 1982); in rage and violent behavior in both the adolescent (Yudofsky et al. 1981) and the elderly; for tension in Type A personalities; and as an adjunct to the neuroleptics in the treatment of schizophrenia (Freedman et al. 1982). Clonidine, the centrally acting alpha-2 blocker, is used to suppress narcotic withdrawal symptoms as well as states of anxiety (Lipman and Spencer 1978; Gold et al. 1980).

Clonidine is particularly interesting because it is known to block alpha-2 receptors in the locus coeruleus, where the highest concentrations of brain norepinephrine are found. Furthermore, Redmond (1977) has deduced from electrical and pharmacological studies that activation of the locus coeruleus produces fear-associated behaviors and increased norepinephrine turnover, while pharmacological inhibition leads to reduction in such behaviors. Clonidine, an alpha-2 adrenergic which passes the blood brain barrier, is known to inhibit locus coeruleus activity.

Methodology

Of the Vietnam combat veterans diagnosed as having the chronic forms of post-traumatic stress disorder according to DSM-III criteria, 12 received propranolol and nine received clonidine.

All have been followed over a six-month period. The clinical follow-up was centered upon the constant symptoms of the condition. Thus we targeted irritability, explosiveness, hyperalertness, intrusive thinking of combat, repetitive nightmares of combat, and sleep, as well as general subjective assessment of personality functioning. At the end of the six-month period all subjects were requested to assess changes on a four-point scale of none, a little, some, and much, and also to comment on their general sense of being since taking the medication.

Prior to commencement of treatment and again at termination, each patient was given a brief assessment of psychosocial status with presenting symptoms. All patients were requested to advise of side effects noticed during the treatment period. Propranolol initially was prescribed in doses of 10 mg to be taken with meals during the day and before bed. At weekly intervals the individual doses were raised by 10 mg until the patients were taking between 120 and 160 mg daily. Clonidine was prescribed initially at 0.1 mg twice daily and then at weekly intervals was raised by 0.1 mg. The maximum dose prescribed to one individual was 0.4 mg and the mean was 0.2 mg.

Results

Of the 12 men on propranolol, 11 reported a positive change in self-assessment at the end of the six-month period. Comments given were: "I'm more relaxed." "I can think better." "I can control my anger." "I don't get upset." "I don't blow." "It's calmed me down." "I'm trying to give things a go." "I had a defeated attitude before." "I have felt the best since my return from Vietnam." "My nerves are calmer." "I have a sense of well being." "I don't feel short-circuited." "I don't feel wired."

As to the response to the specific symptoms, 11 of 12 reported lessened explosiveness, 11 of 12 fewer nightmares and dreams, 9 of 12 improved sleep, 10 of 12 less intrusive thoughts of combat, 7 of 12 lessened startle, and 6 of 12 lessened hyperalertness. Eight of the 12 reported evidence of improvement in psychosocial adaptation. This was evident in better performance on the job, improvement of work at college or school, avoidance of alcohol, increased avocational interest, and lessened pain. The patient who reported the least response to propranolol was also the individual with the greatest psychopathology—suffering a severe catetenoid reaction. Side effects were few in the dosage administered. One patient reported lessened sexual pleasure, another difficulty maintaining an erection, and a third uncertainty about potency. One reported some "lightheadedness," and another patient complained of cloudiness in thinking.

Clonidine was prescribed in doses from 0.2 to 0.4 mg with the majority receiving 0.3 mg daily. Eight of nine patients assessed themselves more positively in terms of their capacity to control their emotions. Typical comments were: "I have a much firmer grip on things." "More control of my emotions and reaction." "I can regulate myself." "I work more easily." "I don't have restlessness." "My dreams are not as long and when I wake up my heart is not beating." "I'm no longer hyper." "I can look at myself." "My fingernails have grown back." "I feel a lot better." "I can control myself." "I'm working and I can go back to school."

As to symptomatic change, eight of nine patients reported lessened explosiveness, seven lessened dreams and nightmares, six better sleep, and four each lessened startle, intrusive thinking, and hyperalertness. All had symptomatic improvement. As to psychosocial improvement, four returned to work and one discontinued alcohol. It is interesting that six of those treated with clonidine had accompanying chronic physical disorders.

Two individuals started on inderal are not included in this assessment. One, a manic depressive, terminated the drug; the other, with a painful mutilating wound, required both tylox and doxepin for pain as well. The first reported he felt more relaxed; the second initially the same. Neither wished to terminate the drug.

Discussion

Prior to the clinical trials of the adrenergic blocking agents, the majority of our patients who were receiving medication were placed on a tricyclic antidepressant. These drugs generally provided improvement in duration of sleep, reduction of depressive affect, and some alleviation in psychosomatic symptoms. However, the general enhancement of self-perception and self-assertion such as has been observed with propranolol and clonidine was never noticed. The repetitive and frightening combat nightmares still occurred, and records of change in intrusive thinking of war experience continued. Men receiving both antidepressants and the adrenergic blockers were engaged throughout in ongoing stress group therapy. Some with serious problems of depression with guilt and violent reactions to the loss of buddies or involvement in atrocities also were seen weekly in individual treatment. This treatment preceded the trials of adrenergic blockers without markedly modifying self-perceptions nor the targeted symptoms followed here.

Our impression is that a well-designed clinical pharmacological research study is in order. Such a study would assess more variable dosage levels as well as compare antidepressants and anxiolytic drugs coupled with physiological assessments to determine if the abnormal arousal patterns are blocked.

As an addendum, we also reported trials of inderal and clonidine in conjunction with tricyclics, neuroleptics, and lithium not included in this study. Clonidine has been prescribed with neuroleptics in two patients without untoward effects. These trials were made in individuals with associated personality disorders, depressed or manic, or schizoid types. Our general impression is that usage of the adrenergic blocking agents attenuates the intensity of symptoms dependent upon somatization of the affects of rage, fear, and anxiety. To alleviate symptoms of guilt and shame, both psychotherapy and sociotherapy remain a necessity.

References

Dobbs D, Wilson WP: Observations on the persistence of war neurosis. J Nerv Ment Dis 21:40–46, 1960

Freedman R, Kirch D, Bell J: Clonidine treatment of schizophrenia: double blind comparison to placebo and neuroleptic drugs. Acta Psychiatr Scand 65:35, 1982

Freud S: Introduction to psychoanalysis and the war neuroses (1919), in Complete Psychological Works, standard ed, vol 17. Translated and edited by Strachey J. London, Hogarth Press, 1959

Gold MS, Pottush AC, Sweeney DR, et al: Opiate withdrawal using clonidine. JAMA 243:343–346, 1980

Kardiner A, Spiegel H: War Stress and Neurotic Illness. New York, Paul B Hoeber, 1947

Kolb LC, Mutalipassi LR: The conditioned emotional response: a subclass of the chronic and delayed post-traumatic stress disorder. Psychiatric Annals 12:979–987, 1982

Lipman JJ, Spencer PS: Clonidine and opiate withdrawal. Lancet 2:521, 1978

Neftel KA, Adler RH, Kappeli L: Stage fright in musicians: a model illustrating the effect of beta blockers. Psychosom Med 44:461–469, 1982

Redmond DE: Alterations in the function of the nucleus coeruleus: a possible model for studies of anxiety, in Animal Models in Psychiatry and Neurology. Edited by Hanin I, Usdin E. Oxford, Pergamon Press, 1977, pp 293–295

Yudofsky S, Williams D, Gorman J: Propranolol in the treatment of rage and violent behavior in patients with chronic brain syndromes. Am J Psychiatry 138:218–220, 1981

7

Post-Traumatic Stress Disorder in the Vietnam Veteran: A Brain-Modulated, Compensatory Information-Augmenting Response to Information Underload in the Central Nervous System?

Augustin de la Pena, Ph.D.

7

Post-Traumatic Stress Disorder in the Vietnam Veteran: A Brain-Modulated, Compensatory Information-Augmenting Response to Information Underload in the Central Nervous System?

CURRENT MODEL OF THE GENESIS OF PTSD IN THE VIETNAM VETERAN

The etiology of post-traumatic stress disorder (PTSD) in the Vietnam veteran is generally viewed in a behavioristic-associationist theoretical framework (Horowitz 1976; Kramer, in press; Brende 1982), central to which are two main assumptions:

1. Behavior is considered to be a passive response to stimuli from "outside" the organism, i.e., behavior, including health-related behavior, is shaped in the main by outside influences that have met the organism in the past: Pavlov's classical conditioning, Skinner's instrumental conditioning, Freud's early childhood experience, and so on; and
2. The natural state of the organism is that of rest, i.e., every stimulus is a disturbance of equilibrium. Behavioral response is geared toward reestablishment of equilibrium, gratification of needs (biological, preeminently hunger and sex), or relaxation of tensions.

Dualism and reductionism are other obsolete ontologic and epistemologic assumptions guiding contemporary research on PTSD. These assumptions have been reviewed and critiqued by von Bertalanffy (1967), Battista (1977), Engle (1977), and de la Pena (1978, 1982). The general theme underlying previous conceptualizations is that the central nervous system (CNS) hyperarousal induced by the uncertain Vietnam combat environment generates an exacerbated state of organismic stress characterized by autonomic hyperarousal and by subsequent defensive perceptual and behavioral strategies (e.g., numbing of behavioral response, withdrawal from the environment) to attenuate the high levels of combat-induced CNS activation. Extant models differ in their explanations of the temporal delay in expression of the stress syndrome. Most, however, assume that elicitation of previously suppressed PTSD symptomatology occurs with the perception of an environmental cue which resembles, or is subjectively associated with, some element(s) of the Vietnam combat experience.

In this chapter, I review some recent psychophysiologic data from my own study of PTSD in Vietnam veterans that is clearly nonsupportive of the current etiologic model and assumptions guiding current work in the area. I show how my data, when combined with a set of principles and assumptions derived from contemporary cognitive psychology, neuroscience, and psychophysiology, point to a radically new view of PTSD etiology.

SYNOPSIS OF RECENT PSYCHOPHYSIOLOGIC STUDY

I recently studied (de la Pena 1983b) various sleeping and waking psychophysiologic parameters in 12 drug-free Vietnam veteran patients (mean age 34.8, age range 29–42) given the diagnosis of PTSD by hospital staff using criteria from the third edition of the *Diagnostic and Statistical Manual of Mental Disorders* (DSM-III) (American Psychiatric Association 1980). Patients were given a structured interview in which they also self-rated various aspects of their waking mood and personally prior to, during, and after their time in Vietnam.

Patients slept two consecutive nights in the lab, from which were computed mean values for traditional sleep parameters (de la Pena 1982). Waking psychophysiologic parameters included pre- and post-sleep resting levels of electroencephalographic, electromyographic and, electro-oculographic activity, as well as systolic and diastolic blood pressure, heart rate, and sublingual temperature.

The majority of patients (from two-thirds to three-fourths, depending on the dependent variable under consideration) gave evidence of the following psychophysiologic profile. Prior to their Vietnam experience, most considered themselves as having low thresholds for the experience of boredom, which to some extent they mitigated by engaging the environment in a very active and extroverted manner. Most apparently had little recourse to "internal" sources of stimulation; i.e., dream recall was highly infrequent, as was the use of imagery and fantasy. Although all patients considered many aspects of their combat experience to be repugnant, most described their Vietnam experience in generally positive terms, stating that the uncertainty of the environment enabled them to experience interest and a sense of competence under stressful circumstances. Six of the patients indicated a strong interest in reenlisting in similar conflagrations and/or the desire to participate again in similar life-threatening environments. Upon return from Vietnam, all described deterioration of psychophysiologic function, an increase in dream (particularly nightmare) recall, and a general feeling of ennui, depression, and anxiety.

Self-rated boredom and Sensation Seeking Scale scores indicated significantly higher values for the PTSD group relative to an age-matched control insomniac population (de la Pena 1983b). Three-fourths of the PTSD group reported the experience of relaxation to be enhanced by vigorous perceptual-motor activity and/or by self-administration of CNS-stimulating drugs (e.g., caffeine, nicotine, marijuana, amphetamines). Moreover, half of the group reported the experience of increased anxiety upon past administration of major and/or minor CNS depressant drugs.

Waking psychophysiologic recordings indicted that most physiologic subsystems showed relatively low levels of activation relative to expected values for age norms, with a minority of subsystems in the high range. Relative to age norms, sleep psychophysiologic recordings indicated long sleep latencies, significantly shorter latencies to the first rapid eye movement (REM) sleep period, depressed deep sleep, and lower sleep efficiency. Three-fourths of the group showed unusually high REM density during REM sleep, and a reverse first night effect (sleep efficiency is higher the first night than on the second night, which is the reverse of the usual pattern). Sleep patterns thus closely resemble those found in primary depression (de la Pena 1978, 1982).

Taken by themselves, the above findings are clearly nonsupportive of the currently favored hyperarousal model of PTSD in Vietnam veterans. Taken in conjunction with the following set of basic principles derived from contemporary cognitive psychology, neuroscience, and psychophysiology, a new view of PTSD etiology in Vietnam veterans is suggested.

CONCEPTUAL SKELETON OF DEVELOPMENTAL-STRUCTURAL APPROACH

Detailed exposition of the following principles of CNS function can be found in some recent publications (de la Pena 1978, 1982, 1983a). One important principle is that increments in experience with stimulus configurations and events build up cognitive (cortical) structures which, in turn, organize subsequent "experience(s)" in related environmental contexts. The building up of cognitive structure results in the construction of cognitive models of expectancies about aspects of stimuli one is likely to encounter in one's moment-to-moment environment. The nervous system apparently works on the principle that unexpected stimuli are processed as "information" in the mathematical sense of the term, while expected stimuli do not provide information, since the "information" is already encoded in the brain's structural and memorial processes.

Any environmental circumstance that provides an accelerated rate of information flow for the brain (e.g., learning new material in school or having to identify quickly informative elements during combat experience) thus has the effect of building up increasingly sophisticated and comprehensive cognitive programs for information processing and/or information reduction. That is, out of necessity for survival, the brain experiencing a surfeit of information flow must construct increasingly efficient programs for information processing in order to maintain information flow rates within tolerable limits. Construction of new cognitive (cortical) models enhances the selective destruction of irrelevant, redundant information, with greater processing of information considered to be relevant for the task at hand (as in solution of a math problem in school, or in the business of survival in a combat environment).

Organisms which have accumulated more experience, then, are construed to have more efficient cognitive models that distinguish informative from uninformative elements in the environment. In ordinary stimulus conditions, they may be conceptualized to be in a state not unlike sensory deprivation, because they have modeled their environments comprehensively and there is little surprise value upon exposure to ordinary stimulus configurations and/or stimulus events.

A second principle is that activity in the CNS and its subsystems works very much like a rubber band. That is, temporary increases in CNS activity (the stretch of the rubber band) brought about by an increase in the information processing demands on the organism (e.g., exercise, paying attention to a novel, unexpected stimulus), are followed by a homeostatic "rebound" decrease in CNS activity (release of the rubber band) to levels below the prestimulus level. These rebound homeostatic changes have been observed in virtually all CNS subsystems studied to date, including electroencephalogram (EEG) (Das and Gastaut 1957), electrocardiogram (EKG) (Wenger and Bagchi 1961), blood pressure (Gellhorn 1957), gross motor behavior (MacLean and Ploog 1962; cf. Oswald 1962, Chapter 9, for review), as well as in other CNS-modulated systems (Brady 1958, 1962).

A third principle is that the brain has a variety of hierarchically organized but imperfectly coupled information-processing controls through which it may actively effect homeostatic changes in its own information input. This occurs when the amount of information processed from the environment falls outside the optional range/rate associated with organized perceptual-cognitive-behavioral function and the experience of relaxation. It is a biologic fact that the cerebral cortex of the brain is equipped to reduce the impact of excessive sensory stimulation, either nonspecifically or selectively (Dawson 1958; Galin 1965; Silverman 1967). Similarly, the brain has protective mechanisms which provide "turning-on" or "augmenting" information-processing responses (e.g., hallucinations, delusions, hyperactivity) when the environment provides an excessively low amount of stimulation or information. These also operate during sleep, with reciprocity of sensory information flow across the states of wakefulness and sleep indicated (de la Pena 1973, 1978, 1982).

CONCEPTUALIZATION OF THE ETIOLOGY OF PTSD

Some Assumptions for Theory Building

The remainder of this chapter will adopt a provisional definition of activation/arousal that is congruent with the generally accepted notion of the nervous system as an information processing system. I will assume that (1) "level of arousal" in a given physiologic subsystem is highly related to the rate of information processing (bits/second) in the subsystem (Pribram 1967); and (2) there is an "overall" information processing rate in the CNS which is highly correlated with the "sum" of the information processing rated in the various hierarchically organized information-processing subsystems in the CNS (John 1976; Battista 1978).

A Psychophysiologic Model of PTSD-VV Etiology

Figure 1 depicts my model of PTSD-VV etiology. Parasympathetic-dominant individuals are posited to have a relatively greater risk for subsequent development of PTSD. That is, prior to participation in the information-rich Vietnam combat environment, the predisposed PTSD parasympathetic-dominant individual is considered to experience a relatively low rate of information flow in the CNS when in ordinary day-to-day sensory environments relative to autonomically balanced or sympathetic-dominant individuals. This is because the parasympathetic-dominant CNS habituates more quickly (Meulders 1962) to sensory information than his autonomically more balanced and/or sympathetic-dominant counterparts. For the former, the information flow rate in the CNS upon exposure to ordinary sensory environments and/or to a resting, quiescent state of motor activity is thus at the (normal) lower end of the range of information flow associated with organized perceptual, cognitive, and behavioral function and the experience of relaxation.

One consequence of this relatively low rate of information processing in a resting, nonstimulated state is an attempt by the understimulated brain to augment its own information flow rate to a higher rate that is more conducive to the experience of relaxation and for organized perceptual, cognitive, and behavioral function, by initiating behaviors (including perceptual and motor behaviors) which augment information flow rates for the CNS,

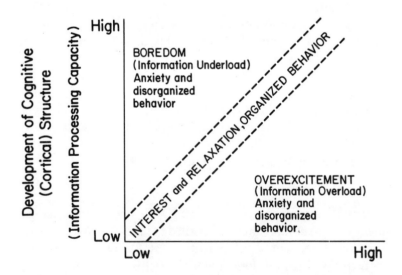

Figure 1 Conceptualization of the Etiology of PTSD-VV

e.g., a vigorous, dynamic, extroverted life style. A primary problem then, for the parasympathetic-dominant individual with a
high risk for subsequent development of PTSD is the experience
of boredom in relatively ordinary, habituated-to, sensory environments.

Owing primarily to one's genetic constitutional physiologic
makeup (i.e., parasympathetic dominance), the individual at risk
for subsequent development of PTSD is able to tolerate the
combat-associated uncertainty and high sensory information load
better than autonomically balanced or ergotropic-dominant individuals (Figure 1). This is because the relatively rapid habituation
rates to sensory stimuli frees up a larger amount of spare cortical
channel capacity to handle the high rates of information flow
associated with the uncertain combat situation. As depicted in
Figure 1, combat experience is posited to increase sensory information flow rate in the CNS of at-risk PTSD individuals, from pre-
Vietnam combat levels that are marginally within the optimal
rates associated with organized psychophysiologic function, to
rates that are comfortably within the optimal rate associated with
organization of psychophysiologic function and the experience of
interest and relaxation. (In this vein, the French philosopher Sartre
[1972] remarked that he had never felt so free as during the war
when, as a member of French Resistance, he was likely to be
arrested and shot at any time.)

However, following return from Vietnam (Figure 1), the at-risk
parasympathetic-dominant individual experiences a rapid "rebound" descent of CNS information flow to levels significantly
below the optimal range associated with organized psychophysiologic function and the experience of interest and relaxation. The
rebound descent is more steep, and the level of CNS information
flow to which the patient falls is lower, relative to autonomically
balanced and ergotropic-dominant individuals; this is because
there is a greater degree of parasympathetic activity which has
been inhibited by the sympathetic autonomic-enhancing effects
of the stimulating, uncertain combat environment. In the absence
of the stimulating combat environment, the high degree of
inhibited parasympathetic activity is released and rebounds to a

very high level, driving information flow rates to aberrantly low levels.

Prior discussion pointed out that the nervous system behaves very much like a rubber band. Using the rubber band analogy, individuals who develop PTSD are considered as very thick rubber bands with a high resistance to "stretch" or CNS excitation. Stretching of the tight, thick rubber band (by the enhanced sympathetic activation associated with the uncertain, stimulating Vietnam combat sensory environment), followed by a release of the rubber band (the individual leaves the uncertain stimulating Vietnam combat environment), is associated with a greater resilience (rebound to levels approximating the nonstretched state) of the highly stretch-resistant rubber band, relative to rubber bands having less resistance to stretch (i.e., individuals with normal autonomic balance and/or individuals characterized by sympathetic dominance).

Another way of thinking about the phenomenon is the following: Individuals who have been exposed to the highly uncertain, sensory information-rich combat environment must develop increasingly more efficient and comprehensive cognitive structures for processing information in order to survive. Not unlike enrolling in a accelerated academic class in which one must develop new cognitive-cortical structures, the Vietnam combat experience is conjectured to have built up in the brains of veterans increasingly comprehensive, efficient programs for handling information. The building up of increasingly efficient information-processing cortical programs has the effect of changing the preferred rate of information processing to a higher level relative to preferred levels prior to the Vietnam experience. That is, increments in experience and/or the development of cognitive structure have the effect of lowering the amount-rate of sensory information processed from ordinary environments, since much of the information already is encoded in structural and/or memorial brain processes. Increments in experience thus necessitate a more active engagement with the environment (i.e., a higher preferred rate of information processing) to rectify the relatively low rates of information flow obtained by experienced cognitive structures upon exposure to ordinary environments and/or activities. Therefore, I posit that when many such parasympathetic-dominant individuals returned home to relatively ordinary sensory environments, they experienced a condition not unlike sensory deprivation accompanied by severe boredom/depression.

This is particularly true of Vietnam veterans as compared to other veterans of previous wars, because Vietnam veterans were largely ignored by society, and their generally lower socioeconomic standing precluded access to educational or interesting vocational pursuits to help fill the information-processing void left by their extrication from the sensory-rich, uncertain Vietnam combat environment. I posit that CNS activation levels and/or information-processing rates in PTSD individuals reached some critical lower limit, thereby calling into play brain-controlled, homeostatic information-augmenting mechanisms to help rectify the brain's own information underload state.

I view certain aspects of the symptomatology in PTSD as the expression of a cortically modulated, information-augmenting mechanism(s), which attempts to rectify an aberrantly low level/rate of information flow in the CNS associated with a powerful rebound of excessive parasympathetic activity in parasympathetic-dominant individuals. Certain aspects of symptomatology in PTSD—nightmares, difficulty in sleep initiation and maintenance, pain syndromes, paranoia (hyperresponsivity to certain environmental stimuli), impulsive-aggressive behavior, and so on—are posited to be the expression of maladaptive information-augmenting mechanisms by which the understimulated, bored brain attempts to rectify its aberrantly low information flow rates to higher, more intermediate levels associated with organized perceptual-cognitive-behavioral function and the experience of interest.

This conceptualization may help to order some of the sleep psychophysiology findings reported earlier. High density REMs and relatively short latencies to REM sleep (as also reported recently in PTSD by Hellekson, [1983]) may be the expression of a sleep sensory information flow control process by which the understimulated, bored (depressed) waking brain helps to rectify its own aberrantly low levels of information flow. That is, the brain gets into the highly exciting, sensory information-rich REM periods more quickly than normal, and it processes an enhanced amount of sensory information per unit of time (as indexed by REM density). In our laboratory, nightmare reports were invariably associated with high density REM periods. Reverse first night effects were obtained because the chronically bored and anxious brain would find that the uncertainty and/or information provided during the first night in the unfamiliar laboratory environment provided increments in information flow to bring CNS information flow rates to within the optimal rate/range associated with the experience of interest and relaxation, which promotes sleep. Difficulty in sleep initiation occurred because the bored, understimulated brain effected a relatively high level of information flow (phenomenologically: anxiety) that was too high for sleep onset, because the brain attempted to rectify the lack of information by increasing its own level of somatic (electromyogram, behavioral) activity. Difficulty in sleep maintenance occurred because high density REMs, normally occurring after five to seven hours of sleep in normal sleepers, occurred as early as the first or second REM period in PTSD patients, and are interpreted by the brain as a signal of sleep satiety (Aserinsky 1969).

The hypothesis of a constitutionally influenced parasympathetic dominance factor predisposing to the development of PTSD also helps to order study findings of paradoxical responses to CNS stimulants (relaxation) and CNS depressants (anxiety) among Vietnam veterans with PTSD. That is, CNS stimulants apparently rectify the aberrantly low levels of information flow in parasympathetic-dominant individuals (associated with relative disorganization of psychophysiologic function and the experience of anxiety) to higher, more intermediate levels associated with organization of function and the experience of relaxation. The paradoxical response to CNS depressants would occur because CNS depressants theoretically would exacerbate an already excessively low level of information flow. The consequence is an increase in anxiety because the brain has an optimal range/rate of information flow associated with organized psychophysiologic function and the experience of relaxation.

The proferred model also predicts that PTSD patients will show intra-interindividual differences in sleep profiles (REM latencies, densities, reverse first night effect, etc.) depending upon the modulation of other cortically controlled, compensatory, information-augmenting mechanisms. For example, during temporal intervals in which waking information flow increases to extremely high levels as a consequence of the brain's effecting hallucinations, delusions, and/or behavioral hyperactivity for itself, it is likely that the amount of endogenous sensory information flow associated with REM sleep (and indexed by measures of phasic REM density, REM sleep latency, etc.) will be low, relative to temporal intervals in which the understimulated brain is mainly employing sleep-associated and/or less drastic waking sensory information-augmenting mechanisms such as mild hypertension and/or mild anxiety to help rectify the information underload. It also seems likely that perceptual and behavioral information-*reducing* controls (numbing of response to the environment) would be called into play when optimal CNS information flow rates are exceeded by the initiation of these gross, information-augmenting mechanisms.

In this view, the development of mild hypertension and/or anxiety in some previously hypotensive PTSD individuals could be interpreted as the expression of a cortically controlled mechanism whereby the understimulated, bored brain augments its own rate of waking *sensory* information processing. Hernandez-Peon (1964) and Silverman (1967) were the first to suggest how such increases in blood pressure might serve to effect an ideal form of psychological defensiveness. That is, increases in blood pressure effect inhibitory control over thought centers of the brain; sensory reactivity is simultaneously facilitated. Because the brain has a limited capacity to process information, enhanced processing of *sensory* information implies depressed processing of *cognitive-ideational* information, hence effecting defense against psychologically disturbing cognitions. Since a reciprocal relation apparently obtains between sensory information flow across the states of wakefulness and sleep (de la Pena 1973, 1978), the enhanced sensory information flow during waking effected by increases in blood pressure and/or anxiety would be associated with a decrease in the intensity of REM sleep-associated sensory information flow (i.e., with a lengthening of the latency to the first REM period and a decrease in REM density) relative to pre-hypertension or pre-anxiety levels, but not as severe a decrement in REM sleep-associated sensory information flow as would obtain with initiation of more powerful sensory information-augmenting processes such as hallucinations and delusions accompanied by hyperactive, explosive and violent behavior.

References

American Psychiatric Association: Diagnostic and Statistical Manual of Mental Disorders, 3rd ed. Washington, DC, American Psychiatric Association, 1980

Aserinsky E: The maximal capacity for sleep: rapid eye movement density as an index of sleep satiety. Biol Psychiatry 1:147, 1969

Battista JR: The holistic paradigm and general system theory. Gen Syst 22:65-71, 1977

Battista JR: The science of consciousness, in The Stream of Consciousness. Edited by Pope KS, Singer JL. New York, Plenum, 1978, pp 55-87

Brady JV: Psychophysiology of emotional behavior, in Experimental Foundation of Clinical Psychology. Edited by Bachrach AJ. New York, Basic Books, 1962, pp 47-63

Brady JV, Porter RW, Conrad DG, et al: Avoidance behavior and the development of gastroduodenal ulcers. J Exp Anal Behav 1:69-72, 1958

Brende JO: Electrodermal responses in post-traumatic syndromes: a pilot study of cerebral hemisphere functioning in Vietnam veterans. J Nerv Ment Dis 170:352-361, 1982

Das NN, Gastaut H: Variations de l'activite electrique du cerveau, du couer et des muscles squelettiques au cours de la meditation et de l'extase yoqique. Electroencephalogr Clin Neurophysiol (Suppl) 6:211–219, 1957

Dawson GD: The effect of cortical stimulation on transmission through the nucleus in the anaesthetized rat. J Physiol 142:210–230, 1958

de la Pena A, Zarcone V, Dement WC: Correlation between measures of the rapid eye movements of wakefulness and sleep. Psychophysiology 10:566–573, 1973

de la Pena A: Toward a psychophysiologic conceptualization of insomnia, in Sleep Disorder: Diagnosis and Treatment. Edited by Williams RL, Karacan I. New York, John Wiley & Sons, 1978, pp 101–143

de la Pena A: The Psychobiology of Cancer: Automatization and Boredom in Health and Disease. South Hadley, Mass, Bergin & Garvey, 1982

de la Pena A: Automatization of sensory information processing: some consequences for perception and behavior, in General Systems Theory and The Psychological Sciences, vol 2. Edited by Gray W, Fidler J, Battista J. Seaside, Calif, Intersystems Publishers, 1983a, pp 59–74

de la Pena A: Sleep and waking psychophysiology of PTSD. Paper presented at Annual meeting of the American Psychiatric Association, New York, May 3, 1983b

Engle GL: The need for a new medical model: a challenge for biomedicine. Science 196:129–136, 1977

Galin D: Background and evoked activity in the auditory pathway: effects of noise shock-pairing. Science 149:761–763, 1965

Gellhorn E: Autonomic Balance and the Hypothalamus. Minneapolis, University of Minnesota Press, 1957

Hellekson C: REM sleep abnormality in a patient with posttraumatic stress disorder. Paper presented at Annual Meeting of the Association of Sleep Disorder Centers, Anaheim, Calif, October 22, 1983

Hernandez-Peon R: Psychiatric Implications of neurophysiological research. Bull Menninger Clin 28:165–185, 1964

Horowitz MJ: Stress Response Syndromes. New York, Jason Aronson, 1976

John ER: A model of consciousness, in Consciousness and Self-Regulation: Advances in Research, vol 1. Edited by Schwartz GE, Shapiro D. New York, Plenum, 1976, pp 1–50

Kramer M, Kinney L, Scharf M: Sleep in delayed-stress victims. Sleep Res (in press)

MacLean PD, Ploog DW: Cerebral representation of penile erection. J Neurophysiol 25:29–55, 1962

Meulders M: Etude Comparative de la Physiologie des Voies Sensorielles Primaires et de Voies Associatives. Brussels, Editions Arscia SA, 1962

Oswald I: Sleeping and Waking: Physiology and Psychology. Amsterdam, Elsevier, 1962

Pribram KH: The new neurology and the biology of emotion: a structural approach. Am J Psychiatry 22:830–838, 1967

Sartre J: quoted in Wilson C: New Pathways in Psychology. New York, Taplinger, 1972, p 27

Silverman J: Variations in cognitive control and psychophysiological defense in the schizophrenias. Psychosom Med 29:225–251, 1967

Von Bertalanffy L: Robots, Men and Minds. New York, George Braziller, 1967, pp 8–9

Wenger MA, Bagchi BK: Studies of autonomic functions in practitioners of yoga in India. Behavioral Sci 6:312–323, 1961

Post-Traumatic Stress Disorder as a Biologically Based Disorder: Implications of the Animal Model of Inescapable Shock

Bessel van der Kolk, M.D.
Helene Boyd, Ph.D.
John Krystal
Mark Greenberg, Ph.D.

8

Post-Traumatic Stress Disorder as a Biologically Based Disorder: Implications of the Animal Model of Inescapable Shock

After a certain moment you just keep running the hundred yard dash. You are always ready for it to come back. I spend all my energy on holding it back. I have to isolate myself to keep myself from exploding. It all comes back, all the time. The nightmares come two, three times a week for awhile. Then they let up for a bit. You can never get angry, because there is no way of controlling it. You can never feel just a little bit. It is all or nothing. I am constantly and totally preoccupied with not getting out of control.

—A Vietnam Veteran

Kardiner (1959) first described the full syndrome of post-traumatic stress disorder (PTSD) on the basis of his observations of World War I (WWI) veterans. He included five principal features of PTSD: (1) persistence of startle responses and irritability, (2) proclivity to explosive reactions, (3) fixation on the trauma, (4) constriction of the general level of personality functioning, and (5) atypical dream life. He described post-traumatic stress as a "physioneurosis," a mental disorder with both psychological and physiological components. Freud (1920) earlier had suggested that traumatic neurosis entails a "physical fixation" to psychic trauma because of the persistence of traumatic memories and dreams.

Grinker and Spiegel (1945) detailed some of the physical concomitants of acute post-traumatic stress, describing myriad autonomic and extrapyramidal symptoms in traumatized combat soldiers, such as masked facies, decreased eyeblink, cogwheel rigidity, coarse tremor of hands and lips, postural flexion, propulsive gait, mydriasis, and gastric distress—in short, many symptoms suggestive of acute central nervous system (CNS) catecholamine depletion.

The post-traumatic symptoms of hyperalertness, hyperreactivity to stimuli, and traumatic reexperiencing form the greater part of the formal criteria from the third edition of the *Diagnostic and Statistical Manual of Mental Disorders* (DSM-III) for the diagnosis of post-traumatic stress disorder. The remaining features of PTSD—such as feelings of estrangement and detachment and constricted affect—can be understood as compensatory symptoms, as illustrated in the quote of the Vietnam veteran at the beginning of this chapter.

Starting with Pavlov (1927), chronic changes in autonomic nervous system activity level in response to repeated traumatic exposure have been demonstrated in both animals and men. Autonomic arousal in people with prior exposure to situations of utter helplessness is liable to be interpreted subjectively as a recurrence of a helpless state with its concomitant fight/flight or surrender responses (Strian and Kliepera 1980). In PTSD it appears that habituation to the traumatic stimulus itself occurs, but that hyperreactivity to associated stimuli persists in the form of startle reactions and flashbacks.

THE MODEL OF INESCAPABLE SHOCK

Perhaps the best available animal model for PTSD involves exposure of animals to inescapable shock. Exposure to inescapable and unavoidable aversive events has widespread behavioral and physiological consequences in animals. Animals that have been actively prevented from escaping severe physical stress such as electric shock, loud noise, or submersion in cold water later show (1) deficits in learning to escape from novel aversive situations,

(2) a decrease in motivation to learn new contingencies, and (3) chronic evidence of subjective distress. The impression that these animals have "given up" has led to the term "learned helplessness" (Maier and Seligman 1976).

The similarity between the behavioral sequelae to inescapable shock in animals and the constricted affect, decreased motivation, and decline in occupational functioning in people after massive psychic traumatization is striking. Thus, the model of inescapable shock provides a unique animal model for a psychiatric condition in humans. Not only does it provide models for behavioral manipulation to reverse the effects of inescapable shock, it also has given insights into the central neurochemical changes which accompany traumatization.

INFLUENCE ON CATECHOLAMINE SYSTEMS

In animals, exposure to inescapable shock increases norepineph-rine (NE) turnover, increases plasma catecholamine levels, depletes brain NE, and increases 3-methoxy-4-hydroxyphenylglycol (MHPG) production (Anisman et al. 1979a, 1979b, 1981). Anisman and others (1981) found that shocks which had no measurable effects on naive animals produced NE depletion and escape deficits in mice previously exposed to inescapable shock. In addition, following inescapable shock, brain dopamine (DA) and serotonin are decreased, and acetycholine is increased (Anisman 1978). While the evidence for NE depletion in mediating the escape deficits has been established most firmly, dopamine appears to play a role in escape and avoidance behavior by means of its effect on the organism's capacity to initiate a response (Fibiger et al. 1975). Thus, it appears that after inescapable shock there is a "chronic and exaggerated neurochemical change in response to subsequent stressors which interferes with response initiation and maintenance" (Anisman 1978).

STRESS-INDUCED ANALGESIA

Another phenomenon observed in inescapable shock experiments with relevance to PTSD in humans is stress-induced analgesia:

Animals exposed to inescapable shock develop analgesia when reexposed to a subsequent stressor within a brief period of time (Maier et al. 1980). While a serotonin mediated short-term analgesic response also exists (Bodner et al. 1978), it is clear that the analgesic response to repeated or prolonged exposure to inescapable stress is mediated by endogenous opioids, and that this response is readily reversible by naloxone (Maier et al. 1980; Willes et al. 1981).

Experimental data show that there is an endorphin response in reaction to inescapable shock in animals, and that repeated exposure to inescapable shock leads to analgesia. Furthermore, data suggest that stress-induced analgesia becomes a conditioned response that eventually occurs after even relatively mild stressors (Maier et al. 1980).

"ADDICTION" TO THE TRAUMA

In clinical reports about people exposed to catastrophic events there are numerous references to a lifelong preoccupation with repetition of the trauma. One example is the observation that children who have been abused have a tendency to provoke and even seek subsequent abuse (Lynch and Roberts 1982; Green 1978). Many concentration camp survivors and veterans with posttraumatic stress disorder seem to place themselves voluntarily in situations reminiscent of the trauma. (Popular culture has demonstrated this powerfully in such movies as *The Pawnbroker*, in the Russian roulette sequences in *The Deerhunter*, and in the opening scene of *Apocalypse Now*.) It is not unlikely that reexposure to traumatic situations in humans evokes a CNS opioid response analogous to that seen in animals in response to inescapable shock. Verebey (1978) claims that opioids, including endogenous opioid peptides, have the following psychoactive properties: (1) anxiolytic or tranquilizing action, (2) reduction of rage and aggression, (3) reduction of paranoia and feelings of inadequacy, and (4) antidepressant action. Historically, opioids have been thought to serve as self-medication for painful or overwhelming affects and related psychopathology.

The parallels between the symptoms of opiate withdrawal and

the hyperreactivity in post-traumatic stress disorder are striking. Jaffe and Martin (1980) list the following for opiate withdrawal: anxiety, irritability, explosive outbursts, insomnia, hyperalertness, and emotional lability. Parallel symptoms of PTSD as listed in DSM-III are hyperalertness, startle responses, difficulty falling asleep, anxiety, and unpredictable explosions of aggressive behavior. We postulate that these parallel symptoms of PTSD and opioid withdrawal have a common etiology, namely central noradrenergic (CNA) hyperactivity in response to a relative decrease in endogenous opioids.

The symptoms of opiate withdrawal are thought to be mediated in part by noradrenergic hyperactivity (Redmond & Krystal 1984), and opiate withdrawal symptoms have been effectively treated with clonidine, an alpha-2 adrenergic agonist (Gold et al. 1982). Recently, Kolb and others (see chapter 6) found clonidine useful in treating the hyperreactivity in PTSD as well.

In summary, based on neurochemical changes in animals exposed to inescapable shock, we postulate that both the central noradrenergic system and CNS opioid peptides play an active and reciprocal role in the initiation and maintenance of post-traumatic stress states. In PTSD, reexposure to trauma may produce an endogenous opioid peptide response which may be experienced subjectively as a sense of control. Subsequent cessation of the traumatic stimulus may produce symptoms of opiate withdrawal such as hyperreactivity, anxiety, and explosive behavior. Thus, trauma seeking in PTSD sufferers may be seen as an attempt to gain a subjective sense of control over overwhelming emotions and physical sensations while simultaneously ensuring a persistence of the intrusive and hyperreactive symptoms of PTSD.

FIXATION ON THE TRAUMA

Intense stimulation of noradrenergic neurons in the CNS has been shown to result in "long-term potentiation" and an enhanced retention of information (Delaney et al. 1983). We postulate that the hypermnesia in post-traumatic stress is due to massive noradrenergic activity at the time of the trauma. In chapter 5,

Kramer demonstrated that autonomic arousal is accompanied by a recurrence of traumatic memories. It is likely that changes in autonomic arousal at night are at least partly responsible for the replicative traumatic nightmares so common in PTSD (van der Kolk et al. 1984).

IMPLICATIONS FOR TREATMENT

If one assumes that the animal model of inescapable shock has parallels with post-traumatic stress disorder in humans, then findings about the reversibility of the effects of inescapable shock in animals may have applications for the treatment of PTSD. First of all, in animals the occurrence of escapable shock prior to inescapable shock attenuates helplessness responses, including analgesia. This may parallel the recurrent observation (Lidz 1946; Moses 1978; Krystal 1978) that people with disrupted early attachment bonds, who thus had prior familiarity with feelings of helplessness, are more likely to develop PTSD than those with more stable backgrounds. Krystal has pointed out that "The occurrence of psychic trauma in a person's past may predispose him to respond excessively and maladaptively to intense affects, resulting in a feeling of being dead or in a variety of dissociative reactions, from depersonalization to psychosis (Krystal 1978).

Second, a variety of psychopharmacological agents, including clonidine (Weiss et al. 1976), benzodiazepines (Sherman and Petty 1980), tricyclic antidepressants (Petty and Sherman 1980), and monoamine oxidase (MAO) inhibitors (Weiss 1975) have been shown to decrease the long-term effects of inescapable shock in animals. While carefully controlled psychopharmacological studies of the treatment of PTSD are lacking, preliminary evidence seems to indicate that clonidine (see chapter 6 of this volume), MAO inhibitors (Hogben and Cornfield 1981), benzodiazepines, and lithium (van der Kolk 1983) may be able to attenuate the severity of PTSD symptoms. The need for carefully controlled psychopharmacological studies for the treatment of hyperarousal states, nightmares, and anhedonia in PTSD is obvious. This research area has suffered greatly from the lack of recognition of

PTSD as a legitimate psychiatric syndrome, and the continued skepticism among many psychiatric researchers about whether the symptoms of PTSD are indeed caused by massive adult psychic trauma, and not the result of an affective disorder, characterological problems, or just malingering.

Teaching an animal previously exposed to inescapable shock to escape subsequent shock by dragging him across into a nonelectrified area will result in the animal trying to escape subsequent shock, and it will reverse at least some of the neurochemical changes caused by inescapable shock (Seligman et al. 1968). If this can be applied to human beings with PTSD it means that if a person with PTSD can reexperience the fact that one's fate is at least partially contingent upon one's actions there will be an attenuation of post-traumatic symptoms. This may mean that the therapist will have to perform the psychotherapeutic equivalent of dragging an animal across a grid to ameliorate the chronic sense of helplessness and victimization which is so common to people with PTSD. The relative effects of psychotherapy and pharmacology on PTSD and their interactions remain a totally unexplored territory.

The treatment implication of the model of addiction to the trauma is very complex. If reliving the trauma is followed by massive anxiety, a conditioned endorphin release, and subsequent withdrawal hyperreactivity, bringing back memories of the trauma in a psychotherapeutic setting might actually increase trauma-seeking behavior as well as anxiety and explosive outbursts of anger. Uncovering psychotherapy would thus lead to clinical deterioration. On the other hand, as we stated in chapter 2, if there can be a working through of the trauma, this can only occur during the phase in which affect is available for psychotherapeutic work. Both Horowitz (1976) and our group found that such affect was available only when memories of the trauma were not totally repressed. The "phase-oriented" treatment model suggested by Horowitz strikes a balance between initial supportive interventions to minimize the traumatic state and increasingly aggressive "working through" at later stages of treatment. Systematic desensitization is another relatively unexplored, but promising area of treatment.

Conclusions

The role of psychological trauma as the precursor of mental disorders has been a much neglected area of research ever since Freud abandoned his theory of actual seduction as the origin of hysteria. We now know again that the defense mechanism of repression and dissociation of affect and cognition are common sequelae to traumatic events. Psychological trauma may be a precursor of such diverse psychiatric syndromes as psychosomatic conditions, chronic pain syndromes, and certain borderline conditions, as well as adult post-traumatic stress disorder.

Attempts to fit the sequelae of psychic trauma into neat psychodynamic or behavioral models have proven to be quite unsatisfactory. Although the human experience of overwhelming helplessness is infinitely more complex than exposing an animal to inescapable electric shocks, the ability to measure neurochemical changes in traumatized animals allows psychiatrists a unique opportunity to assess the physiological consequences of events with clear psychopathological sequelae. The full implications of the animal data on the consequences of inescapable shock remain to be explored.

References

Anisman H: Neurochemical changes elicited by stress: behavioral correlates, in Psychopharmacology of Aversively Motivated Behavior. Edited by Anisman H, Bignami G. New York, Plenum, 1978

Anisman HL, Sklar LS: Catecholamine depletion in mice upon reexposure to stress: mediation of the escape deficits produced by inescapable shock. J Comp Physiol Psychol 93:610–625, 1979

Anisman HL, Grimmer L, Irwin J, et al: Escape performance after inescapable shock in selectively bred lines of mice: response maintenance and catecholamine activity. J Comp Physiol Psychol 93:229–241, 1979b

Anisman HL, Ritch M, Sklar LS: Noradrenergic and dopaminergic interactions in escape behavior: analysis of uncontrollable stress effects. Psychopharm Bull 74:263–268, 1981

Bodnar RJ, Kelly DD, Glusman M: Stress induced analgesia: time course of pain reflex alterations following cold winter swims. Bull Psychonomic Soc 11:333–336, 1978

Delaney R, Tussi D, Gold PE: Long-term potentiation as a neurophysiological analog of memory. Pharmacol Biochem Behav 18:137–139, 1983

Fibiger HC, Zis AP, Phillips G: Haloperidol-induced disruption of conditioned avoidance responding: attenuation by prior training or by anticholinergic drugs. Europ J Pharm 30:309–322, 1975

Freud S: Beyond the pleasure principle (1920), in Complete Psychological Works, standard ed, vol 18. Translated and edited by Strachey J. London, Hogarth Press, 1959

Gold M, Pottash AC, Sweeney D, et al: Antimanic, antidepressant and antipanic effects of opiates: clinical, neuroanatomical and biochemical evidence. Ann New York Acad Sci 140–150, 1982

Green AH: Self-destructive behavior in battered children. Am J Psychiatry 135(5):579, 1978

Grinker RR, Spiegel JJ: Men Under Stress. New York, McGraw-Hill, 1945

Hogben GL, Cornfeld RB: Treatment of traumatic war neurosis with phenelzine. Arch Gen Psychiatry 38:440–445, 1981

Horowitz MJ: Stress Response Syndromes. New York, Jason Aronson, 1976

Jaffe JH, Martin W: Narcotic analgesics and antagonists, in Pharmacological Basis of Therapeutics, 6th ed. Edited by Gilman AG, Goodman LS, and Gilman A. New York, Macmillan, 1980

Kardiner A: Traumatic neurosis of war, in American Handbook of Psychiatry. Edited by Areti S. New York, Basic Books, 1959

Krystal H: Trauma and affects. Psychoanal Study Child 33:81-116, 1978

Lidz T: Nightmares and the combat neuroses. Psychiatry 9:37-49, 1946

Lynch M, Roberts J: Consequences of Child Abuse. New York, Academic Press, 1982

Maier SF, Seligman MEP: Learned helplessness: theory and evidence. J Exp Psychol [Gen] 105:3-46, 1976

Maier SF, Davies S, Grau JW: Opiate antagonists and long-term analgesic reaction induced by inescapable shock in rats. J Comp Physiol Psychol 94:1172-1183, 1980

Moses R: Adult psychic trauma: the question of early predisposition and detailed mechanisms. Int J Psychoanal 59:353-363, 1978

Pavlov IP: Conditioned Reflexes: An Investigation of the Physiological Activity of the Cerebral Cortex (1927). Edited and translated by Anrep, GV. New York, Dover, 1960

Petty F, Sherman AD: Reversal of learned helplessness by imipramine. Communications in Psychopharmacology 3:371-373, 1980

Redmond DE Jr, Krystal JH: Multiple mechanisms of withdrawal from opioid drugs. Ann Rev Neurosci vol 7, (in press)

Seligman MEP, Maier SF, Geer J: The alleviation of learned helplessness in the dog. J Abnorm Psychol 73:256-262, 1968

Sherman AD, Petty F: Neurochemical basis of the action of antidepressants on learned helplessness. Behav Neural Biol 30:119-134, 1980

Strian F, Kliepera C: Die Bedeutung psychoautonomer reaktionen fur entstehung und persistenz von angstzustanden. Nervenarzt 49:576-583, 1980 van der Kolk BA: Psychopharmacological issues in post-traumatic stress disorder. Hosp Community Psychiatry 34:683–691, 1983

van der Kolk BA, Blitz R, Burr WA, et al: Nightmares and trauma. Am J Psychiatry 141:187–190, 1984

Verebey K, Volavka J, Clouet D: Endorphins in psychiatry. Arch Gen Psychiatry 35:877–888, 1978

Weiss JM, Glazer HI, Pohorecky LA, et al: Effects of chronic exposure to stressors on subsequent avoidance-escape behavior and on brain norepinephrine. Psychosom Med 37:522–524, 1975

Weiss JM, Glazer HI, Pohorecky LA: Coping behavior and neurochemical changes: an alternative explanation for the "learned helplessness" experiments, in Animal Models in Human Psychobiology. Edited by Serban G, Kling A. New York, Plenum Press, 1976

Willes J, Petren J, Cambier J: Stress-induced analgesia in humans: endogenous opioids and naloxone reversible depression of pain reflexes. Science 212:689–690, 1981